CCM
Practice Questions

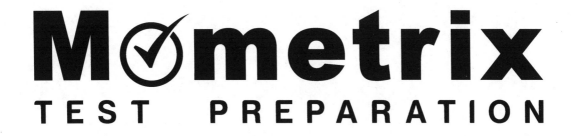

DEAR FUTURE EXAM SUCCESS STORY

First of all, **THANK YOU** for purchasing Mometrix study materials!

Second, congratulations! You are one of the few determined test-takers who are committed to doing whatever it takes to excel on your exam. **You have come to the right place.** We developed these practice tests with one goal in mind: to deliver you the best possible approximation of the questions you will see on test day.

Standardized testing is one of the biggest obstacles on your road to success, which only increases the importance of doing well in the high-pressure, high-stakes environment of test day. Your results on this test could have a significant impact on your future, and these practice tests will give you the repetitions you need to build your familiarity and confidence with the test content and format to help you achieve your full potential on test day.

Your success is our success

We would love to hear from you! If you would like to share the story of your exam success or if you have any questions or comments in regard to our products, please contact us at **800-673-8175** or **support@mometrix.com**.

Thanks again for your business and we wish you continued success!

Sincerely,
The Mometrix Test Preparation Team

TABLE OF CONTENTS

Practice Test #1

1. The FOCUS (find, organize, clarify, uncover, start) performance improvement model to facilitate change is primarily used to:

    a. Develop solutions.
    b. Evaluate outcomes.
    c. Identify problems.
    d. Implement programs.

2. A situation that requires termination of case management includes:

    a. The client is uncooperative with case management plan.
    b. The client has met maximum allowable benefit for case management.
    c. The client's cost of care exceeds that projected.
    d. The client has failed to meet goals and expected outcomes.

3. The primary function of the case manager is:

    a. Coordination of care.
    b. Quality management.
    c. Cost management.
    d. Outcomes management.

4. In order to qualify for Medicare based on a 63-year-old spouse's work record, the applicant must be at least:

    a. 62 years old.
    b. 63 years old.
    c. 64 years old.
    d. 65 years old.

5. The SAFE questions to ask a client suspected of being a victim of abuse include questions about Stress/Safety, Afraid/Abused, Friends/Family, and:

    a. Escalation.
    b. Emergency plan.
    c. Employment.
    d. Education.

6. In motivational interviewing, *change talk* refers to:

    a. Instructions provided by the interviewer.
    b. A statement of goals by the client.
    c. Statements indicating commitment to change.
    d. A summarizing statement of client's progress.

7. The most important factor in cost management is:

    a. Purchasing in bulk and limiting choices in equipment and supplies.
    b. Conducting cost comparisons and choosing the least expensive options.
    c. Providing the minimal care necessary to achieve acceptable outcomes.
    d. Eliminating duplication of services and care fragmentation.

8. The agency that provides guidelines and staff training for case managers related to transitions of care is:

    a. Commission on Accreditation of Rehabilitation Facilities (CARF).
    b. Utilization Review Accreditation Commission (URAC).
    c. American Institute of Outcomes Care Management (AIOCM).
    d. Agency for Healthcare Research and Quality (AHRQ).

9. A rehabilitation center that has received accreditation from the Commission on Accreditation of Rehabilitation Facilities (CARF) indicating the need for improvement in case management must submit a Quality Improvement Plan (QIP) within:

    a. 30 days.
    b. 60 days.
    c. 90 days.
    d. 120 days.

10. The primary focus of job analysis is on the specific requirements of the:

    a. Job.
    b. Person.
    c. Company.
    d. Law/Regulations.

11. In order for an organization to receive health plan accreditation from the National Committee for Quality Assurance (NCQA), the organization must report and meet measures of performance that are divided into 6 standards of focus. These standards include all of the following EXCEPT:

    a. Outcome evaluation.
    b. Member experience.
    c. Population health management.
    d. Network management.

12. A client covered by the Civilian Health and Medical Program of the Department of Veterans Affairs (CHAMPVA) would need preauthorization for:

    a. Durable medical equipment (purchase cost of $1,000 or more).
    b. Referral to specialists.
    c. Diagnostic procedures.
    d. Hospice services.

13. The National Quality Forum's CMS readmission measures cover all of the following EXCEPT: heart attack, heart failure, and pneumonia,

    a. Pulmonary embolism.
    b. Heart attack and heart failure.
    c. Pneumonia.
    d. COPD and knee/hip replacement.

14. Case management information systems (CMISs) generally include:

    a. Financial management programs.
    b. Standardized plans of care.
    c. Computerized physician order entry systems.
    d. Pharmacy information systems.

15. *Failure to rescue* refers to:

    a. Inability to identify life-threatening complications in time to prevent death.

    b. Failure to identify clients in abusive situations.

    c. Failure to prevent death in clients who experienced severe trauma.

    d. Inability to prevent a client from experiencing a psychotic break.

16. The primary goal of community-based case management is:

    a. Assist clients to meet personal goals.

    b. Coordinate services to ensure optimal outcomes and prevent hospitalization.

    c. Assist clients to access services to promote independent functioning.

    d. Provide care in the most cost-effective manner.

17. A hospice case manager is primarily responsible for:

    a. Providing emotional support to the dying and family members.

    b. Ensuring that costs related to care are minimized.

    c. Ensuring dying clients remain in their home rather than in a hospital.

    d. Coordinating services to provide care and comfort to the dying.

18. The TRICARE program that utilizes a preferred provider organization (PPO) is:

    a. TRICARE Standard.

    b. TRICARE Extra.

    c. TRICARE Prime.

    d. TRICARE Reserve Select.

19. The Blaylock Risk Assessment Screening Score (BRASS) is a tool used to:

    a. Identify older adults at risk of prolonged hospitalization.

    b. Assess risk of falls in hospitalized clients.

    c. Identify clients at risk for hospital-acquired infections.

    d. Assess the client's ability to provide self-care on discharge.

20. In order to consult effectively with a client and family about client needs, the first step is to:

    a. Outline possible interventions.

    b. Establish a trusting relationship.

    c. Identify desired outcomes.

    d. Evaluate the client's/family's resources.

21. If a caregiver keeps a client with moderate dementia heavily sedated so that the client sleeps most of the day, this is an example of:

    a. A safety measure.

    b. Neglect.

    c. Psychological abuse.

    d. Physical abuse.

22. The appropriate referral for a client with swallowing problems following a stroke is:

    a. Occupational therapist.

    b. Speech therapist.

    c. Physical therapist.

    d. Nutritionist.

23. The primary goal of a work hardening program is for the client to:
    a. Increase strength and mobility.
    b. Evaluate the need for job modifications.
    c. Return to full work.
    d. Determine the degree to which a client can return to work.

24. For a client covered by Medicare A for rehabilitation hospitalization, the admission functional independence measure (FIM) scores must be obtained during the first:
    a. 24 hours.
    b. 48 hours.
    c. 3 calendar days.
    d. 5 calendar days.

25. When transferring a client from a bed to a chair, the proper transfer technique to use with a cooperative client able to bear only partial weight and having almost no upper body strength is:
    a. Stand and pivot technique.
    b. Powered standing assist with 1 caregiver.
    c. Seated transfer aid.
    d. Full body sling lift with 2 caregivers.

26. A client who qualified for 18 months of COBRA coverage as a beneficiary and was determined by Social Security to be disabled 40 days after beginning coverage and remained disabled for the entire 18 months is entitled to a total of:
    a. 18 months of coverage.
    b. 29 months of coverage.
    c. 36 months of coverage.
    d. 48 months of coverage.

27. A client who would have been eligible for Medicaid in January but does not apply until June first is entitled to coverage that starts: *(confirm accuracy of answer explanation)*
    a. January 1.
    b. June 1.
    c. March 1.
    d. May 1.

28. To prevent back injury when standing on the floor and lifting heavy items, the items should be:
    a. 30 to 40 inches above the floor.
    b. At waist level.
    c. At knee level.
    d. 20 to 30 inches above the floor.

29. An indigent uninsured client with a medical emergency must be provided care at:
    a. Any private physician's office.
    b. Any emergency department.
    c. Any public hospital.
    d. Free clinics only.

30. A person who was injured on the job and unable to work for 3 months would receive Workers' Compensation benefits at the level of:

    a. Permanent total disability (PTD).
    b. Temporary partial disability (TPD).
    c. Permanent partial impairment (PPI).
    d. Temporary total disability (TTD).

31. In order to qualify for Supplemental Security Income (SSI), the maximum limit for resources for a married couple is:

    a. $1,000.
    b. $2,500.
    c. $3,000.
    d. $4,000.

32. Allowing a person to start work 2 hours earlier to accommodate a radiation treatment schedule is an example of:

    a. Job modification.
    b. Job restructuring.
    c. Work hardening.
    d. Job analysis.

33. In utilization management, an example of misutilization is:

    a. Inappropriate admission.
    b. Inadequate diagnostic testing.
    c. Inappropriate length of stay.
    d. Treatment error.

34. With the accelerated rapid-cycle change approach to quality improvement, the team members focus on:

    a. Analysis.
    b. Solutions.
    c. Problems.
    d. Work flow.

35. A cost-containment strategy in which all clients receiving similar services or treatments from the same provider have the same payment rate is:

    a. Episode-of-care payments.
    b. Performance-based provider payments (P4P).
    c. All-payer rate setting.
    d. Global payments.

36. The most common strategy used to contain pharmaceutical costs is:

    a. Use of generic drugs.
    b. Use of preferred drug lists.
    c. Volume purchasing of drugs.
    d. Use of mail order prescriptions.

37. Before receiving benefits, the client with a preferred provider organization (PPO) insurance plan may have to pay:
   a. A copayment.
   b. The deductible.
   c. The premium only.
   d. The deductible and a copayment.

38. In order to meet the *recent work test* for Social Security Disability Insurance (SSDI), a client who becomes disabled in the quarter when he turns 30 years old must have worked:
   a. 1.5 years out of the previous 3-year period.
   b. 3 years out of the previous 5-year period.
   c. 4.5 years out of previous 9-year period.
   d. 5 years out of the previous 10-year period.

39. An indemnity insurance plan is usually an example of:
   a. HMO.
   b. Fee-for-service.
   c. PPO.
   d. POS.

40. Under Medicare A's inpatient prospective payment system, the organization should expect to be paid according to the payment classification of:
   a. Medicare severity diagnosis-related group (MS-DRG).
   b. Fee-for-service (FFS).
   c. Case-mix group (CMG).
   d. Ambulatory payment category (APC).

41. A pharmacy benefit manager (PBM) is primarily responsible for:
   a. Providing prescription drug plans.
   b. Administering prescription drug plans.
   c. Assisting clients to obtain necessary drugs.
   d. Preventing abuse of drugs.

42. Generally, the most important factor in whether a purchaser profits from a viatical settlement is the:
   a. Length of time the insured lives after purchase.
   b. Original purchase price of the plan.
   c. Monthly payment schedule for the plan.
   d. Face value of the plan on payment of benefits.

43. An individual purchasing an insurance plan through an exchange should expect that a silver tier plan will pay:
   a. 90% of medical expenses.
   b. 80% of medical expenses.
   c. 70% of medical expenses.
   d. 60% of medical expenses.

44. Under Medicare Part A and/or Part B, the home health services that are covered include:
   a.   Homemaker service.
   b.   Round-the-clock care in the home.
   c.   Meals delivered to the home.
   d.   Intermittent skilled nursing care.

45. The percentage of employees who are employed in businesses that offer insurance is the:
   a.   Offer rate.
   b.   Enrollment-when-eligible rate.
   c.   Enrollment rate.
   d.   Eligibility rate.

46. The primary determinant as to whether people enroll in employer-sponsored health coverage is the:
   a.   Wages of the applicant.
   b.   Cost to the applicant.
   c.   Age of applicant.
   d.   Ethnicity and gender of applicant.

47. Resource utilization groups (RUGs) and minimum data sets (MDSs) are used to establish payment rates for:
   a.   Home health agencies.
   b.   Ambulatory client care.
   c.   Acute care hospitals.
   d.   Skilled nursing facilities.

48. The type of managed care plan that allows a client to see physicians and care providers within a network but to seek outside treatment in some circumstances is:
   a.   Health maintenance organization (HMO).
   b.   Exclusive provider organization (EPO).
   c.   Point of service plan (POS).
   d.   Preferred provider organization (PPO).

49. The health maintenance organization (HMO) model that allows individual or groups of physicians to contract with an HMO to provide services while also seeing non-HMO clients is:
   a.   Staff model.
   b.   Independent practice association (IPA).
   c.   Group practice.
   d.   Direct contract.

50. Health insurance is based on the principle of:
   a.   Risk management.
   b.   Risk reduction.
   c.   Risk avoidance.
   d.   Risk pooling.

51. A client who is temporarily disabled and has short-term disability insurance should usually expect to collect:

 a. 100% of pre-disability salary.
 b. 75% of pre-disability salary.
 c. 60% of pre-disability salary.
 d. 50% of pre-disability salary.

52. According to the Americans with Disabilities Act (ADA), public transportation must provide lifts that can accommodate occupied manual or powered wheelchairs that weigh up to a minimum of:

 a. 500 pounds.
 b. 600 pounds.
 c. 700 pounds.
 d. 800 pounds.

53. The government entity that requires that personal protective equipment be readily available at the worksite and in appropriate sizes is the:

 a. CDC.
 b. FDA.
 c. OSHA.
 d. CMS.

54. The FDA will allow emergency use of a drug with filing of an Investigational New Drug (IND) exemption for:

 a. One disease/condition only.
 b. One client only.
 c. No more than 4 clients.
 d. A 1-month time period only.

55. Under the Health Insurance Portability and Accountability Act (HIPAA) regulations, clients who request copies of laboratory results must receive them within:

 a. 24 hours.
 b. 48 hours.
 c. 14 days.
 d. 30 days.

56. The CMS Clinical Quality Measures, in their Adult Recommended Core Measures, recommend that screening for depression (NQF 0418) begin at age:

 a. 12 years.
 b. 14 years.
 c. 18 years.
 d. 21 years.

57. When screening the body mass index (BMI) as part of the CMS core measure, what is the acceptable BMI range for a 55-year-old?

 a. 18.5-25.
 b. 18.5-28.
 c. 20-30.
 d. 23-30.

58. The best solution for working with a client who expresses extreme prejudice toward ethnic minorities and the LGBT population is to:

    a. Tell the client his attitude is reprehensible.
    b. Refuse to work with the client.
    c. Provide professional service and avoid debate.
    d. Provide minimal service and avoid interacting with client.

59. The government agency that provides clinical guidelines and recommendations for health care professionals is:

    a. CDC.
    b. NIH.
    c. AHRQ.
    d. CMS.

60. The primary purpose of a benchmark study is to identify:

    a. Best practices.
    b. Gaps in performance.
    c. Cost-saving measures.
    d. Areas for further research.

61. When conducting client needs assessment as part of caseload calculations, the most important factors are:

    a. Acuity, personal/family psychosocial issues, and environment.
    b. Diagnosis, personal psychosocial issues, and length of stay.
    c. Acuity, age, and environment.
    d. Diagnosis, mental status, and functional ability.

62. The primary purpose of predictive modeling is to:

    a. Develop an effective model of care.
    b. Predict hospital length-of-stay and need for care.
    c. Increase cost-effectiveness of client care.
    d. Identify clients at risk for negative outcomes.

63. The purpose of a concurrent review of a hospitalized client is to assess:

    a. The client's medical necessity for admission.
    b. The need for prescribed treatments.
    c. The need for continued hospitalization.
    d. The client's need for discharge planning.

64. As part of utilization management, the Milliman Care Guideline that is appropriate for clients with complex clinical situations and diagnoses for which a specific guideline does not exist is:

    a. General recovery.
    b. Chronic care.
    c. Inpatient and surgical care.
    d. Ambulatory care.

65. **Focused utilization management programs that target only specific client populations often result in:**
    a. Cost savings and improved care.
    b. Care deficiencies.
    c. Skewed data and inaccurate interpretation of data.
    d. Time and cost savings.

66. **Under the hospice benefit for end-of-life care, *home* is defined as:**
    a. The client's primary residence.
    b. The client's primary residence or a skilled nursing facility.
    c. Any place the client is residing.
    d. The client's primary residence or any licensed health care facility.

67. **A core indicator of end-stage disease is:**
    a. Serum albumin <2.5 g/dL.
    b. Difficulty swallowing.
    c. Increased medical complications.
    d. Significant dyspnea, even with oxygen.

68. **The term that refers to a case manager's area of practice or knowledge is:**
    a. Function.
    b. Role.
    c. Venue.
    d. Domain.

69. **The case manager expects that a client with a Karnofsky Performance Status Scale score of 30 will require:**
    a. No special intervention.
    b. Occasional assistance with personal care.
    c. Institutional or hospital care.
    d. Frequent assistance with personal care.

70. **A client's case management plan should focus on:**
    a. Determining needed resources.
    b. Establishing goals and prioritizing needs.
    c. Identifying strategies for care and interventions.
    d. Providing cost-effective care.

71. **A discharge planning evaluation must include an evaluation of the:**
    a. Client's need for post-hospitalization services.
    b. Projected costs of post-hospitalization services.
    c. Community agencies available.
    d. Client's cognitive abilities.

72. **The primary purpose of admission certification is to determine:**
    a. The correct diagnostic-related group (DRG) for the client.
    b. The client's maximal insurance benefit.
    c. The client's projected cost for hospitalization.
    d. The medical necessity of admission.

73. The case manager should always avoid:

    a. Working extended hours with one client.

    b. Dual relationships with clients.

    c. Working in more than one role.

    d. Empathizing with clients about their conditions.

74. If a person who identifies herself as the client's wife calls and asks for information about a hospitalized client, the case manager should:

    a. Provide the information the person requests.

    b. Make arrangements to meet with the client and spouse.

    c. Ask the person questions about the client to verify identification.

    d. Give out no information about the client.

75. The case manager may break a client's confidentiality:

    a. Under no circumstances.

    b. When a client is in need of emergent care.

    c. When the client fails to follow the case management plan.

    d. When the client fails to keep an appointment.

76. An appropriate statement for a case manager to make on a social networking site about working with clients is:

    a. "I really like some of my clients, especially the older woman who calls me 'dear.'"

    b. "I had a client today who threw a screaming fit at me."

    c. "I have to see way too many clients in a day!"

    d. No statement whatsoever.

77. The best tool to combat fear of technology and data is:

    a. Education.

    b. One-on-one supervision.

    c. Clear structure.

    d. Consultant.

78. To increase compliance, the case manager who institutes changes in procedures in order to improve patient outcomes should include:

    a. Penalties.

    b. Supervision.

    c. Accountability.

    d. Raw supportive data.

79. The factor that has the most significant effect on hospital length of stay is:

    a. Age.

    b. Comorbidities.

    c. Number of surgical procedures.

    d. Diagnosis.

80. When the client of a mental health case manager refuses case management after being discharged from a mental institution, the case manager should:
- a. Assess the need for court-ordered case management.
- b. Try to convince the client to have case management.
- c. Allow the client to refuse services.
- d. Refer the client to the public health department.

81. When doing financial analysis of diagnosis-related groups (DRGs), *relative weights* refer to value assigned to DRG based on:
- a. Diagnoses only.
- b. Complexity and resources needed.
- c. Estimated length of stay.
- d. Level of care and diagnoses.

82. When doing case management evaluation using the cost-effectiveness analysis method, *sensitivity analysis* refers to:
- a. Determining who pays and who benefits.
- b. Timing of accrual of costs and benefits.
- c. Specifying types of costs.
- d. Testing assumptions and validating conclusions.

83. In assisted living facilities, staffing must include:
- a. 24-hour staffing (skilled or unskilled).
- b. 24-hour skilled nursing.
- c. 12-hour skilled nursing and 12-hour unskilled.
- d. 12-hour staffing (skilled or unskilled).

84. The best placement for a 24-year-old client with schizophrenia being discharged from a psychiatric institution for the first time in 4 years is likely:
- a. Skilled nursing facility.
- b. Private apartment.
- c. Shared apartment.
- d. Group home.

85. The average length of stay in an acute hospital for a client 65 to 84 years of age with septicemia is approximately:
- a. 5 to 7 days.
- b. 8 to 10 days.
- c. 11 to 14 days.
- d. 15 to 20 days.

86. An example of an emergent group is:
- a. Legislative body.
- b. Research team.
- c. Social agency.
- d. Group of friends.

87. A case manager who influences members of a group but is not in turn influenced by the members is exemplifying:

  a. Sequential interdependence.
  b. Mutual, reciprocal interdependence
  c. Unilateral interdependence.
  d. Multilevel interdependence.

88. In dealing with conflict, a staff person who follows the guidelines of the case manager he or she disagrees with is exhibiting:

  a. Accommodation.
  b. Compromise.
  c. Avoidance.
  d. Collaboration.

89. When evaluating research, the *P* value that is most statistically significant is:

  a. 0.01
  b. 0.5
  c. 0.002
  d. 0.04

90. When conducting an interview, the case manager should avoid questions that begin with:

  a. Why.
  b. When.
  c. Where.
  d. How.

91. *Sentinel procedures* refers to:

  a. Procedures that resulted in a client's death.
  b. Procedures associated with life-threatening diseases/conditions.
  c. First procedures carried out on a client.
  d. Procedures that place the client at risk of complications.

92. When making decisions about case management based on catastrophic diagnoses, diagnoses would include:

  a. Pneumonia.
  b. Syncope.
  c. Solid-organ transplants.
  d. Seizure disorder (new onset).

93. The passive acquisition of cases refers to:

  a. Routine acquisition of all of one category of client.
  b. Acquisition based on client request.
  c. Acquisition based on direct observation of need.
  d. Acquisition by referral from health care providers.

94. The best response to a client who is progressing well after a stroke but remains extremely fearful and anxious about discharge is to:

    a. Explore the client's concerns with the client.
    b. Reassure the client that everything will be all right.
    c. Refer the client to a psychologist.
    d. Delay discharge until the client feels ready.

95. The best method of sharing data with staff about the positive outcomes of case management is by providing:

    a. Raw data.
    b. Percentages.
    c. Charts and graphs.
    d. Narrative explanations.

96. When preparing a quality improvement report, the case manager should begin with:

    a. An outline of interventions.
    b. The indicator that was measured.
    c. The type of measurement used for assessment.
    d. The results of the intervention.

97. When completing a cost-benefit analysis, an example of a "soft" cost savings is:

    a. Decreased length of hospitalization stay.
    b. Prevention of complications.
    c. Client's change to a provider in the network.
    d. Transfer from lower level of care.

98. The case manager who wants to justify further intervention for a rehabilitation client who has not met performance goals should begin with:

    a. The data on admission to the program.
    b. Current data related to ability to perform.
    c. An explanation of performance goals.
    d. An overview of benefits allowed for the client in their insurance plan.

99. A client who refuses to talk to the case manager because her husband had a bad experience with a case manager is exhibiting a barrier to communication involving:

    a. Physical interference.
    b. Impaired processing ability.
    c. Psychological impairment.
    d. Perceptions.

100. Prior to the initial interview with a client, the case manager should:

    a. Review the client's medical records.
    b. Interview the client's nursing staff.
    c. Review the client's insurance plan.
    d. Assess the client's ability to pay any necessary costs.

101. When clients have multiple comorbidities and are under the care of multiple physicians, one of the first things the case manager should assess is:

    a. Financial condition.
    b. Psychological status.
    c. Medication reconciliation.
    d. Functional ability.

102. The focus of case management in a pre-acute environment, such as a physician's office or clinic, is often on:

    a. Coordination of providers.
    b. Collaboration.
    c. Utilization.
    d. Prevention.

103. In negotiating prices with an out-of-network health care provider, the case manager should begin by:

    a. Asserting limits to reimbursement.
    b. Researching prices.
    c. Establishing goals for client care.
    d. Appealing to the health care provider's empathy.

104. The primary goal of quality improvement projects is to:

    a. Evaluate where and how medical errors occur.
    b. Assign blame for medical errors.
    c. Determine the need for improvement.
    d. Develop cost-saving processes.

105. The model of acute care case management that follows the client's progress through acute hospitalization to ensure effective, safe, and cost-effective transition from acute care to post-acute care is:

    a. Integrated functions.
    b. Disease management.
    c. Clinical resources.
    d. Outcomes management.

106. In a payer-based case management model, the case manager is generally an employee of the:

    a. Physician.
    b. Agency providing care.
    c. Client.
    d. Insurance company.

107. The most common reasons for screening clients to determine need for case management are:

    a. Diagnosis, high rates of resource utilization, and high costs of care.
    b. Diagnosis, age, and high rates of resource utilization.
    c. Diagnosis, age, and high costs of care.
    d. Diagnosis, high rates of resource utilization, and projected length of stay.

108. A physical disability would include:

a. Blindness.
b. Deafness.
c. Osteoarthritis in knees.
d. Balance disorder.

109. The Chronic Care Model is primarily utilized in the:

a. Client's home.
b. Primary care setting.
c. Skilled nursing facility.
d. Acute hospital.

110. In the Patient-Centered Medical Home Model of care, the team leader coordinating care is usually a:

a. Case manager.
b. Nurse.
c. Social worker.
d. Physician.

111. Palliative care is intended for those who:

a. Have specific diagnoses, such as cancer or heart disease.
b. No longer have curative treatments.
c. Need to improve the quality of life by managing symptoms.
d. Need comfort care during the last 6 months of life.

112. Clients who are receiving physical therapy as part of community rehabilitation through a home health agency and Medicare can expect to receive:

a. 1 to 3 hours of therapy, usually 5 days a week.
b. 30 minutes to 1 hour of therapy, usually 3 days a week.
c. 3 hours of therapy, usually 3 days a week.
d. 3 or more hours of therapy, usually 5 days a week.

113. The case manager realizes that when a client transitions between providers, the client is:

a. At increased risk for complications and negative outcomes.
b. Likely to show continued improvement and less need for care.
c. Likely to have decreased information and participation in care.
d. More likely to ask that case management be discontinued.

114. Statements that outline the level of performance expected of a professional, such as a case manager, are included in:

a. Case management plans.
b. Standards of care.
c. Evidence-based practice guidelines.
d. Standards of practice.

115. In an acute hospital interdisciplinary team, the individual primarily responsible for assessing the post-discharge needs of the client is the:

  a. Physician.
  b. Case manager.
  c. Social worker.
  d. Occupational therapist.

116. In order to qualify for inpatient rehabilitation, a client must be able to undergo rehabilitation therapy for:

  a. At least 3 hours daily for 5 to 7 days per week.
  b. Less than 3 hours daily for up to 5 days per week.
  c. 1 hour of therapy 5 days per week.
  d. At least 5 hours of therapy 5 days per week.

117. A swing bed agreement with CMS allows a hospital to:

  a. Move a client from one room to another.
  b. Place clients in Stryker frames to facilitate change in position.
  c. Use the same bed for acute or skilled nursing facility care.
  d. Have some beds without any type of side rails.

118. Most medical insurance will not cover:

  a. Hospice care.
  b. Skilled nursing care.
  c. Sub-acute care.
  d. Intermediate care.

119. The purpose of health coaching is to:

  a. Teach clients about their diseases.
  b. Help clients achieve their goals.
  c. Teach clients about preventive measures.
  d. Help clients understand their insurance plans.

120. According to the Rancho Los Amigos Levels of Cognitive Functioning tool, a client with a score of VIII is:

  a. Nonresponsive to all types of stimuli.
  b. Confused and agitated.
  c. Exhibiting a localized response to stimuli.
  d. Exhibiting appropriate behavior.

121. The most useful way in which to divide groups of clients is by:

  a. Risk stratification.
  b. Projected costs.
  c. Gender.
  d. Ethnicity/Cultural background.

122. If a $100,000 investment in hiring a case manager results in savings of $120,000, then $20,000 represents the:
    a. Capital gains.
    b. Profit.
    c. Return on investment.
    d Avoidable costs.

123. Disease management programs are usually intended for:
    a. Specific population of clients.
    b. All clients.
    c. Hospitalized clients.
    d. Both low- and high-risk clients.

124. The case manager working with clients with substance abuse usually focuses on assisting clients to:
    a. Benefit from therapy.
    b. Obtain needed resources.
    c. Develop motivation for change.
    d. Avoid hospitalization.

125. When a client tells the case manager that her caregiver does not allow her to use the telephone or read her mail, the case manager should suspect that the client is:
    a. Confused.
    b. Lying.
    c. Experiencing psychological abuse.
    d. Experiencing neglect.

126. A client who is a devoutly religious Catholic and believes her health problems are punishment for sins may benefit most from:
    a. Self-help groups.
    b. Pastoral counseling.
    c. Self-help literature.
    d. Psychotherapy.

127. When doing telephonic case management, the primary focus is usually on:
    a. Cost-effective use of resources.
    b. Answering questions.
    c. Triaging clients.
    d. Authorizing services.

128. A warning sign that a case manager is developing a relationship with a client that is too personal is the case manager:
    a. Enjoying meeting with the client.
    b. Recognizing that the client's values are different from the case manager's.
    c. Feeling attracted to a client but not acting on the attraction.
    d. Asking the client about personal matters unrelated to client's needs.

129. When a client has signed a release of information form so the case manager can provide information to a therapist, the case manager should:
   a. Release all available information.
   b. Ask the client, item by item, what should be released.
   c. Release the minimum information necessary to meet the request.
   d. Edit the information released to the therapist.

130. A terminally ill client who believes that prayer will heal her probably:
   a. Is in a state of denial.
   b. Is delusional.
   c. Depends on faith for comfort.
   d. Needs education about her disease.

131. A bipolar client who is very nervous about transitioning into the community from a sheltered environment may benefit from:
   a. A support group.
   b. A 12-step program.
   c. Antidepressants.
   d. Peer counseling.

132. According to the Transtheoretical Model of change, the process of change that people go through when they express feelings (positive and negative) about change is:
   a. Self-liberation.
   b. Dramatic relief.
   c. Consciousness raising.
   d. Self-reevaluation.

133. In Roberts' Seven-Stage Crisis Intervention Model, the first stage includes:
   a. Assessing lethality.
   b. Establishing rapport.
   c. Identifying major problems/precipitants.
   d. Exploring alternatives.

134. Clients with schizophrenia, depression, or bipolar disease are at high risk for:
   a. Violent behavior.
   b. Impaired mobility.
   c. Seizure disorders.
   d. Dual diagnosis.

135. The Digit Repetition Test is primarily used to diagnose:
   a. Early dementia.
   b. Depression.
   c. Delirium.
   d. Attention deficits.

136. A client who insists that the case manager sit down with the client and explain the health care options in detail and outline them in writing is exhibiting:

  a. Anxiety.
  b. Arrogance.
  c. Self-determination.
  d. Self-advocacy.

137. An elderly low-income home care client who is losing weight because she doesn't like to cook and lives on junk food may benefit most from:

  a. Meal delivery services.
  b. Admission to an assisted living facility.
  c. Referral to a nutritionist.
  d. Homemaker services.

138. If an uninsured client who is ineligible for Medicaid is unable to pay for an expensive chemotherapeutic drug, the initial step to solving the problem is to:

  a. Suggest the client ask the physician about taking a less expensive drug.
  b. Contact the physician to ask if the client can be treated without charge.
  c. Suggest the client conduct a fund-raising campaign.
  d. Determine if the drug company has a pharmaceutical assistance program.

139. RotaCare clinics provide free medical care to:

  a. Clients who are homeless only.
  b. Clients who are uninsured, underinsured, and/or homeless.
  c. Diabetic clients only.
  d. Infants and children only.

140. The case manager who cannot find food or shelter for a homeless client may receive assistance for the client from the local:

  a. Salvation Army.
  b. Public Health Department.
  c. RotaCare clinic.
  d. Medical society.

141. A client who suffers from posttraumatic stress syndrome, which interferes with his ability to work and communicate with others, would be best classified as having:

  a. Mental impairment.
  b. Psychiatric disability.
  c. Psychiatric illness.
  d. Psychological illness.

142. A client who remains grief-stricken and depressed 10 months after her husband's death and has been unable to work or care for her family or home would probably benefit most from a:

  a. Support group.
  b. Psychologist.
  c. Bereavement counselor.
  d. Psychiatrist.

143. Self-directed Medicaid services allows participants to:
   a. Make decisions about all aspects of services.
   b. Apply for Medicaid services over the Internet.
   c. Determine how much financial support they need.
   d. Make decisions over certain specified services.

144. Chronic disease in elderly adults is most often associated with:
   a. Depression.
   b. Dementia.
   c. Substance abuse.
   d. Partner abuse.

145. The instrument that is most appropriate to assess general health and disability across all medical disciplines, including mental, neurological, and substance abuse, is:
   a. Global Assessment of Functioning (GAF) test.
   b. Instrumental Activities of Daily Living (IADL) assessment.
   c. The Time and Change test.
   d. World Health Organization Disability Assessment Schedule 2 (WHODAS-2).

146. A series of steps in treatment based on client response and developed through scientific and evidence-based research in order to standardize a specific type of care is referred to as a(n):
   a. Protocol.
   b. Decision tree.
   c. Algorithm.
   d. Care map.

147. The purpose of the Patient Activation Measure (PAM) is to:
   a. Assess client's health status.
   b. Assess client's ability for self-care.
   c. Identify clients who require interventions.
   d. Determine client's readiness for learning.

148. If a client has not been adhering to the plan of care, the best solution for the case manager is to:
   a. Discontinue case management services.
   b. Notify the client's physician.
   c. Discuss barriers to adherence with the client.
   d. Remind the client of his or her responsibilities.

149. When a client's condition does not progress according to expectations as outlined in the clinical pathway, this is referred to as a(n):
   a. Variance.
   b. Complication.
   c. Error.
   d. Discrepancy.

150. When doing force field analysis to develop an outcomes management program, an example of a restraining force is:

    a. Satisfaction with the status quo.
    b. Desire to predict needed skill sets.
    c. Need to track present and future costs.
    d. Desire to use outcomes as marketing tools.

151. If an insurance company has denied coverage for therapy that the case manager feels should have been covered for a client, the first thing the case manager should do is:

    a. Determine an alternative.
    b. Assist the client to file an appeal.
    c. Ask the physician to call the insurance company.
    d. Call the insurance company directly.

152. If a client was seriously injured at work but feels that the employer was negligent and plans to sue, the client should:

    a. Apply for Workers' Compensation and then file suit.
    b. File suit and then apply for Workers' Compensation.
    c. Wait before making any type of decision.
    d. File suit and avoid applying for Workers' Compensation.

153. A TRICARE beneficiary is eligible for TRICARE for Life if the person has:

    a. Medicare A.
    b. Medicare B.
    c. Medicare A and B.
    d. no Medicare.

154. The billing code that is utilized for services such as ambulance and durable medical equipment is:

    a. ICD-10-CM.
    b. ICD-10-PCS.
    c. CPT-4.
    d. HCPCS-Level II.

155. If the case manager wants to apply the correct diagnostic code for outpatient services to a billing form, the case manager would utilize:

    a. CPT-4.
    b. NDC.
    c. ICD-10-PCS.
    d. ICD-10-CM.

156. The term that would most apply to a transgender female (biological male) who is sexually attracted to females is:

    a. Lesbian.
    b. Gay.
    c. Bisexual.
    d. Heterosexual.

157. A case manager assigned to a population health program in an African American community with high rates of hypertension and diabetes should initially focus education on:

    a. Compliance with treatment.
    b. Diet and exercise.
    c. BP and glucose monitoring.
    d. Drug and alcohol use.

158. The case manager is preparing a client to undergo a functional capacity evaluation required by the client's insurance company following injury and tells the client that the evaluation will not include:

    a. Lifting ability.
    b. Range of motion.
    c. Motivation.
    d. Stamina.

159. If a client with a disability is applying for a job and asks the case manager if he should disclose the disability to the employer, the best response is:

    a. "It's always best to disclose a disability."
    b. "You only need to disclose if you expect an accommodation."
    c. "It's best to never disclose unless asked directly."
    d. "Whatever you feel comfortable doing is fine."

160. If the organization is using the John Hopkins ACG® (Adjusted Clinical Group) system, the case manager expects that it will:

    a. Decrease utilization of case management services.
    b. Provide incentives to decrease the costs of care.
    c. Make predictions based on the practice pattern of the clinician.
    d. Help to predict clients' future health needs.

161. When determining if a client has achieved a healthcare goal, such as lowered blood pressure, the case manager should:

    a. Observe and measure personally.
    b. Ask the client if the goal was achieved.
    c. Review the client's healthcare record.
    d. Consider all aspects of the client's condition.

162. If the case manager is concerned that a client's attention seems to wander, the best test to assess attention is:

    a. Confusion Assessment Method.
    b. Time and Change Tool.
    c. Digit Repetition Test.
    d. Trail Making Test.

163. If a client with COPD has tried repeatedly to quit smoking but feels that quitting is impossible, the case manager should:

    a. Remind the client of the health benefits of smoking cessation.
    b. Provide support and assist the client in establishing short and long-term goals.
    c. Remind the client of the adverse effects of smoking.
    d. Enlist family member is pressuring the client to quit.

164. The primary reason for stratifying risk is to:
a. Save healthcare costs for high risk individuals.
b. Better allocate the case manager's time and resources.
c. Identify red flags that indicate the need for case management services.
d. Provide preventive intervention before problems arise.

165. If the case manager contacts the pharmacist regarding a client's medications and verifies the prescriptions with the physician, this meets the case management goal of:
a. Coordinating care.
b. Improving the quality of care.
c. Encouraging client engagement.
d. Reducing health care costs.

166. During a concurrent review, the case manager should assess whether:
a. Care is medically necessary.
b. The client is receiving an appropriate level of care.
c. The care provided has met client's needs.
d. All healthcare providers are collaborating.

167. If a client in an acute care hospital is stable but will require 7 further days of IV antibiotics during recovery from surgery and a severe post-operative infection, the most appropriate level of care is:
a. Long-term acute care facility.
b. Skilled nursing facility.
c. Subacute care facility.
d. Acute care hospital.

168. If conducting a behavioral health assessment for a client who is noncompliant with treatment, the case manager should focus on:
a. Behavior in the home.
b. Behavior outside the home (work, social gatherings).
c. The effects of behavior.
d. The reason for behavior.

169. Insurance companies hire case managers primarily to:
a. Provide the best care possible.
b. Reduce costs of care.
c. Educate the client.
d. Investigate claims.

170. If a client's insurance is an exclusive provider organization (EPO) and the client chooses to see a physician outside of the network and receives a bill for $500, the client must pay:
a. 20%.
b. 50%.
c. 80%.
d.100%.

171. The client who has been covered by an employer-sponsored insurance plan but is not qualified to apply for COBRA is a:

a. Client who was laid off from work.
b. Client who divorced the primary insurance holder (employee).
c. Client who quit the job that provided the insurance.
d. Widow/Widower of the deceased primary insurance holder.

172. If a client on Medicare requires durable medical equipment, the costs should be covered by:

a. Medicare A.
b. Medicare B.
c. Medicare C.
d. Medicare D.

173. If a client is admitted to a skilled nursing facility (SNF) after a qualifying stay in an acute hospital, Medicare provides coverage for up to:

a. 30 days.
b. 60 days.
c. 100 days.
d. 120 days.

174. In order for a client to qualify for Social Security Disability Insurance (SSDI), the client or the person on whom the client is dependent must have been employed for at least:

a. 5 years.
b. 10 years.
c. 15 years.
d. 20 years.

175. If a Medicare client does not meet the qualifications for SSDI but is 68 years old, low income, and disabled, the case manager should advise the client to apply for:

a. Faith-based charity.
b. Medicaid.
c. TANF.
d. SSI.

176. In order for a client to qualify for VA benefits, the client must have been honorably discharged and served on active duty for a minimum of:

a. 24 months.
b. 36 months.
c. 48 months.
d. 72 months.

177. If a client was injured at work and is undergoing rehabilitation for physical strengthening 2 days a week in preparation for returning to work, this is referred to as:

a. Work hardening.
b. Work conditioning.
c. Work preparation.
d. Work adjustment.

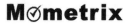

178. To classify inpatients for reimbursement, Medicare utilizes:
- a. MS-DRG.
- b. AP-DRG.
- c. IR-DRG.
- d. APR-DRG.

179. According to Tuckman's stages of group development, the stage in which differences of opinion come to the surface and members begin forming subgroups with those who share similar opinions is:
- a. Storming.
- b. Norming.
- c. Performing.
- d. Mourning.

180. The score for the REALM (Rapid Estimate of Adult Literacy in Medicine) test is based on the:
- a. Number of words the client can define.
- b. Number of questions the client can answer correctly.
- c. Number of words the client can pronounce.
- d. Number of words the client can spell.

Answer Key and Explanations for Test #1

1. C: The FOCUS performance improvement model to facilitate change is primarily used to identify problems. The model is usually used in conjunction with other change models (such as PDCA) to find solutions to the problems. FOCUS:

- *Find*: Review the organization for processes that aren't working well (problems).
- *Organize*: Create a team with people who understand the problem.
- *Clarify*: Use brainstorming to find solutions.
- *Uncover*: Determine the reason the problem has occurred.
- *Start*: Begin the change process.

2. B: A situation that requires termination of case management includes when the client has met the maximum allowable benefit for case management. The case manager should plan in advance for the termination, taking all possible steps to ensure the client's case management plan is adequate and can continue without direct supervision. Other reasons for termination include client wishes, achievement of goals, and a change in health care setting or type/level of care that precludes continued case management.

3. A: While these are four essential functions, the primary function of the case manager is coordination of care. The case manager collaborates with others in the health care team to provide day-to-day care and provide discharge planning as well as education for client and family. The case manager facilitates safe passage through the health care system and plans for appropriate follow-up clinical and community services. Consistent and effective coordination of care helps to promote cost-effective care as well by identifying problems and facilitating early intervention.

4. D: In order to qualify for Medicare based on a 63-year-old spouse's work record, the applicant must be at least 65 years old. The qualifying spouse must be 62 years of age or older. The applicant may also qualify based on the work record of a former spouse or deceased spouse. Those who do not qualify based on their own or their spouse's work record may pay premiums for Part A, Part B, and Part D with payment for Part A prorated according to the applicant's work record.

5. B: The SAFE questions to ask a client suspected of being a victim of abuse include questions about Stress/Safety, Afraid/Abused, Friends/Family, and Emergency plan:

- Stress/Safety: What are your stresses? Do you feel safe?
- Afraid/Abused: Have you or your children been afraid, threatened, or abused, physically or sexually?
- Friends/Family: Do your family and friends know about the abuse? Can you tell them or ask them for support?
- Emergency plan: Do you have resources and a place to go? Do you need help finding shelter now? Do you want to see a social worker or counselor?

6. C: Motivational interviewing aims to help clients resolve their ambivalence about behavioral change. Change talk is an element of motivational interviewing and refers to statements that clients make indicating that they are committed to change. The interviewer's role is to help guide the client toward change talk, as there is a correlation between change talk and successful change in behavior. Change talk may proceed from statements about a desire and need to change to indications of a willingness to take steps to facilitate change.

27

7. D: The most important factor in cost management is eliminating duplication of services and care fragmentation. The case manager may also manage costs by conducting cost comparisons when obtaining supplies and equipment, but the least expensive option is not always the best, so quality is also a consideration. The case manager may exercise creativity and ingenuity in providing services in a cost-effective manner. The case manager may need to actively obtain data in order to show cost-effectiveness and influence coverage by the individual's insurance carrier.

8. B: Utilization Review Accreditation Commission (URAC) provides guidelines and staff training for case managers related to transitions of care, providing both case manager standards and performance measures. *Transitions of care* refer to changes the client encounters in locations, types and levels of care, and care providers. The program reviews the components of case management, methods for engaging customers in education, staff training, assessment and planning, coordination of care, and reporting. Measures include readmissions, worker's compensation, complaint responses, customer satisfaction, refusal of services transitions, and activation.

9. C: Once an organization has completed the application process and received accreditation from the Commission on Accreditation of Rehabilitation Facilities (CARF) indicating the need for improvement in case management or any other aspect, the organization must submit a Quality Improvement Plan (QIP) within 90 days. The QIP should provide a blueprint of plans for improvement or outline steps already taken to remedy the problems highlighted by CARF. CARF provides standards manuals and training to help organizations understand and prepare for accreditation.

10. A: The primary focus of job analysis is on the specific requirements of the job. This detailed analysis may include tasks, as well as time, knowledge, and skills needed to complete tasks. Other aspects include the environment, necessary tools and equipment, and relationships. Job analysis may be used to develop training programs by identifying needs, to determine the degree of compensation for a job, to develop selection procedures, and to perform performance review. Job analysis may include observation, surveys, and interviews.

11. A: In order for an organization to receive health plan accreditation from the National Committee for Quality Assurance (NCQA), the organization must report measures of performance in more than 100 areas. These measures fall under 6 standards: quality management and improvement, population health management, network management, utilization management, credentialing, and member experience. Outcomes evaluation is a subset within the quality management and improvement standard. Accreditation requires a comprehensive initial review and then submission of annual reports.

12. D: CHAMPVA requires preauthorization for hospice services, durable medical equipment with cost of purchase or rental of $2,000 or more, mental health services, substance abuse service, transplants (organ/bone marrow), and dental procedures associated with medical conditions. Diagnostic procedures and referrals to specialists do not require preauthorization if they are medically necessary. CHAMPVA provides health care coverage for spouses and children of disabled veterans or veterans who died in the line of duty. Those eligible for TRICARE are not also eligible for CHAMPVA.

13. D: The National Quality Forum's CMS readmission measures cover heart attack, heart failure, pneumonia, COPD and knee/hip replacement, but do not cover pulmonary embolism. NQF is focusing on reducing readmissions by 10% as a means to improve client care and outcomes and to reduce costs through its All-Cause Admissions and Readmissions Measures project. Studies indicate that approximately 20% of Medicare clients are readmitted to a hospital within 30 days of discharge.

14. B: Case management information systems (CMISs) generally include standardized plans of care to provide treatment protocols that support best practices. CMISs help to identify resources available in order to prevent complications. The systems are able to also identify patterns, variances, and trends among past and present records. If trends are identified, then the system can provide decision support to help with planning and management of care. CMISs are especially valuable for clients with complex needs, such as those who are elderly or have chronic diseases and multiple morbidities.

15. A: Failure to rescue (FTR) is a term used in reporting mortality rates and refers specifically to the inability to identify life-threatening complications in time to prevent death through appropriate interventions. Overall FTR rates have decreased because of fewer postoperative complications, but FTR rates have increased in some areas, such as urologic procedures. Clients at increased risk of FTR include the elderly, clients with severe illness, ethnic minorities, Medicaid clients, and clients at urban hospitals.

16. C: While all of these are important goals, the primary goal of community-based case management is to assist clients to access services in order to promote independent functioning. Community-based case managers must be familiar with health care and service providers in the community and should work closely with an interdisciplinary team, including social workers and appropriate therapists, in order to identify and attend to clients' needs. Clients and family members should be active participants in planning.

17. D: A hospice case manager is primarily responsible for coordinating services to provide care and comfort to the dying and their families. While pain management and emotional support are important elements of case management, and cost-effectiveness is always a concern, hospice clients often have multiple needs, which may include oxygen therapy, wound care, and nutritional support. Caregivers may require respite or assistance, and families may have financial difficulties. The hospice case manager must view the client holistically in order to ensure that the client receives appropriate care and comfort.

18. B: TRICARE Extra utilizes a paid provider organization, so the plan beneficiary receives a 5% discount on copayments. There is no additional charge for selecting this option. TRICARE provides civilian health care benefits for military, retired military, and dependents, as well as some who are in the military reserve. TRICARE is under control of the Defense Health Agency (DHA). TRICARE has a number of programs, including TRICARE for Life, which serves as a supplemental insurance to Medicare, and TRICARE Young Adult, for dependents who have aged out of the TRICARE.

19. A: The Blaylock Risk Assessment Screening Score (BRASS) is a tool used to identify older adults at risk of prolonged hospitalization. These clients are often in need of intense discharge planning, so identifying the clients early allows for the planning process to begin in order to prevent unanticipated post-discharge issues. BRASS contains 10 items related to functional status, abilities, and history. Clients receive scores for each item, with a total score of 10 indicating the need for home care resources, 11-19 indicating a need for intensive discharge planning, and more than 20 indicating at risk for placement other than at home.

20. B: For consultation with a client and family to be effective, the case manager must first establish a trusting relationship. The case manager must begin by cultivating trust at the first visit by being honest, respecting the client's privacy, and persevering in order to establish credibility. The case

29

manager should expect some resistance and testing but must remain nonjudgmental while clarifying the client's perception of issues and determining the effect the client's and family's beliefs, attitudes, and behaviors may have.

21. D: If a caregiver keeps a client with moderate dementia heavily sedated so the client sleeps most of the day, this is an example of physical abuse. While much physical abuse is more obvious, with bruises and physical injuries attesting to beating, kicking, slapping, or pinching, physical abuse also includes such behaviors as forced feeding, using unnecessary physical restraints to limit a client's mobility, and using excessive drugs to control behavior, often so that the caregiver can neglect the client and avoid providing needed care.

22. B: While a stroke client may have the need for multiple therapists, the speech therapist is specifically trained to evaluate and provide therapy for clients with difficulty swallowing. This may include exercises as well as modifications of foods (such as thickening watery liquids). The occupational therapist may assist the client in adjusting to physical limitations and learning to perform activities of daily living. The physical therapist may help to restore strength and mobility while the nutritionist may teach the client about meal planning and dietary needs.

23. C: The goal of a work hardening program is for the client to return to full work. Clients must usually be able to participate for at least 4 hours a day 3 to 5 days per week. Activities may include strengthening and mobility exercises; job practice or job simulation; training regarding safety issues, work pacing, work behaviors, and time management; and evaluation of the need for job modifications. Each client has an individualized plan with measurable goals and objectives.

24. C: For a client covered by Medicare A for rehabilitation hospitalization, the admission FIM scores must be obtained during the first 3 calendar days, and the scores should be based on activities the client performs during the entire 3 days. A 3-day discharge assessment window is also used for the discharge FIM score, but the assessment must be completed within any 24-hour period within those 3 days (except for assessment of bowel and bladder function, which requires 3 days for assistance and 7 days for incontinence).

25. D: The proper transfer technique to use with a cooperative client able to bear only partial weight and with almost no upper body strength is a full body sling lift with 2 caregivers. Because the client lacks upper body strength, the client is unable to assist with the transfer, so other transfer techniques put both the client and the caregiver at risk for injury. Different types of slings are available, including toileting and bathing (mesh) slings.

26. B: A COBRA beneficiary who qualifies for 18 months of COBRA coverage as a beneficiary and is determined by Social Security to be disabled within 60 days of beginning COBRA coverage and who remains disabled throughout the 18-month period of coverage is entitled to apply for an 11-month extension for a total of 29 month of coverage. If a person qualifies for an extension because of disability, all qualified beneficiaries in the family are also eligible to apply for the same extension.

27. C: Coverage can be 3 months retroactive (March 1) if the client would have been eligible if he or she had applied at the earlier time, allowing for coverage of medical expenses incurred prior to application. Clients are eligible for Medicaid if they are younger than 65 years and their income is up to 138% of the federal poverty level. The 100% federal poverty level (for a family of four) in 2019 was $26,200. The Affordable Care Act expanded Medicaid coverage but not all states have opted for expansion, so eligibility requirements and benefits may vary somewhat from state to state.

28. A: To prevent back injury, items to be lifted should be 30 to 40 inches above the floor or the surface the person is standing on. In some cases, people may need to stand on a stool, or table height may need to be lowered. If reaching for items on shelves, the person should use a stepstool or portable steps, making sure that the equipment is appropriate. Work surfaces that are of variable height are ideal but not always available.

29. B: Under the Emergency Medical Treatment and Labor Act (EMTALA), emergency departments are legally required to provide a medical exam and stabilizing care to anyone who seeks care, regardless of the person's ability to pay. Once a client is stabilized, the client may be transferred to another facility, such as a county hospital that takes indigent clients. Various other services may be available to treat indigent clients, such as free clinics, and some hospitals, such as teaching hospitals, may provide free services.

30. D: Temporary total disability (TTD) is paid for the time period when a person is unable to work. Temporary partial disability is paid when a person is able to work part-time but cannot yet resume full-time work. Permanent partial impairment is paid as an addition to regular disability payments if the person has a permanent disability of some type related to the injury, such as amputation of a finger. Permanent total disability is paid when the person is too disabled as a result of the injury to earn a regular income.

31. C: In order to qualify for SSI, the maximum limit for resources for a married couple is $3,000. Resources include cash, savings accounts, stocks and bonds, land, vehicles, personal property, life insurance, and anything else of significant value that be sold. Those who are eligible include those 65 years and older and those who are blind or disabled with limited income and resources. Applicants must be US citizens or within an eligible category of aliens (such as Amerasians and Cubans).

32. A: Allowing a person to adjust work hours to accommodate a treatment schedule is an example of job modification. The actual work stays the same, but modifications are made to allow the person to carry out the necessary tasks. In this case, the hours of work are changed to accommodate treatment. Other examples of work modification include allowing people (such as cashiers) to sit instead of stand while carrying out duties or allowing a person to work fewer hours.

33. D: Utilization management is done to determine if the use of services, facilities, and procedures is appropriate and medically necessary. Utilization management requires analysis of:

- Misutilization: Treatment errors or other inefficient processes, such as scheduling problems
- Overutilization: Inappropriate admissions, inappropriate length of stay, inappropriate levels of care, and inadequate documentation for use of resources (such as diagnostic testing)
- Underutilization: Failure to admit, inadequate diagnostic testing, inadequate levels of care
- Interventions should be planned based on the outcomes of this analysis, considering cost-effectiveness and process improvement strategies

34. B: With the accelerated rapid-cycle change approach to quality improvement, the team members focus on identifying solutions rather than analysis. There are 4 areas of concern in this method:

- Models for rapid-cycle change: Doubling or tripling the rate of quality improvement by modifying and accelerating traditional methods
- Pre-work: Problem statements, graphic demonstrations of data, flowcharts, and literature review. Team members identified
- Team creation: Rapid action (also sometimes rapid acceleration or rapid achievement) teams (RATs) formed
- Team meetings and workflow: Meetings/work scheduled over 6 weeks from initial work to implementation

35. C: A cost-containment strategy in which all clients receiving similar services or treatments from the same provider have the same payment rate is all-payer rate setting. Rates may be set by the provider or by government regulations, such as through Medicaid. The goal is to reduce the high costs of health care and reduce price competition, although the costs to the provider may increase because of the need to negotiate rates and process claims, as reimbursement schedules may vary according to diagnoses or other criteria.

36. A: While all of these strategies are used to contain pharmaceutical costs, the most common strategy is the use of generic drugs rather than brand-name drugs. This strategy alone may save up to 80% of the cost of drugs, depending on the medications and the volume. Pharmacy benefit programs often require a substantially larger copay for non-generic drugs or require the person to pay the entire cost. Prescription forms usually contain a place where physicians can agree to generic substitutions.

37. D: With a preferred provider organization, the client must always pay a deductible, which is a set amount that varies according to the plan but may range from $100 to $5,000 or more. Additionally, many plans now also require a copayment, which may be a percentage of the cost or (more commonly) a set amount, such as $25. With a PPO, clients are expected to see a physician from within a list of preferred providers. Some plans allow clients to seek care outside the PPO, but the clients' share of expenses increases.

38. C: In order to meet the "recent work test" for SSDI, a client who becomes disabled in the quarter when he turns 30 years old must have worked half of the years since the quarter after turning 21, or 4.5 years out of the 9 years that have elapsed. Those who become disabled on or before the quarter of turning 24 must have worked 1.5 years out of the preceding 3 years, and those 31 or older must have worked at least 5 out of the preceding 10 years.

39. B: An indemnity insurance plan is usually a fee-for-service type plan. This type of plan may include a deductible and a copayment, which may vary depending on the cost and type of plan. Fee-for-service plans usually allow clients to choose their physicians, although clients may be limited by the physicians available. The types of preventive services available to clients will also vary. Preventive services are usually exempt from the deductible and may or may not require copayment.

40. A: Under Medicare A's inpatient prospective payment system, the organization should expect to be paid according to the payment classification of Medicare severity diagnosis-related group (MS-DRG). The MS-DRG is determined by the principal and secondary diagnoses (8 or less), ICD-10 procedures (6 or less), client's age, client's gender, and client's discharge status. Various other factors, including the hospital location and cost of living, are used to calculate the hospital-specific prices. Hospitals serving large numbers of low-income clients and teaching hospitals may receive additional payment.

41. B: Pharmacy benefit managers (PBMs) are primarily responsible for administering prescription drug plans, which are provided by insurance companies (such as Blue Cross) or health care systems (such as Kaiser Hospitals). PBMs process and pay claims, maintain the formulary, and establish contracts and discount agreements with pharmacies and drug companies. Examples of PBMs include Express Scripts, United Health, and CVS Caremark. PBMs may provide networks of pharmacies to which clients can go to get drugs as well as mail-order programs that allow clients to obtain 3-month supplies of drugs.

42. A: Generally, the most important factor in whether a purchaser profits from a viatical settlement is the length of time the insured lives after purchase. The purchaser of another's life insurance plan generally tries to pay as far below face value as possible because plans usually require continued monthly payments. Viatical settlements are generally profitable if the covered person dies within 2 years, but if the person lives for 10 to 20 years, then the purchaser may lose money.

43. C: An individual purchasing an insurance plan through an exchange should expect that a silver tier plan will pay 70% of medical expenses. Individually purchased insurance plans are categorized by tiers, indicating the average percentage of medical expenses covered:

- Platinum: 90%
- Gold: 80%
- Silver: 70%
- Bronze: 60%

A "catastrophe" plan is also available for those under age 30 with limited income, but these plans have very limited coverage. Under the Affordable Care Act, insurance plans must cover Essential Health Benefits (EHBs).

44. D: Under Medicare Part A and/or Part B, the home health services that are covered include intermittent skilled nursing care, pathology services (lab testing), occupational therapy, respiratory therapy, physical therapy, and speech-language therapy. Medicare may also cover social services, intermittent home health aide services, and the cost of medical supplies and durable medical equipment. Services that are not covered include homemaker services, round-the-clock care, and home delivery of meals. Additionally, clients must meet specific criteria, such as being homebound and requiring intermittent skilled nursing care (for other than drawing of blood for lab tests).

45. A: Enrollment rates associated with insurance:

- Offer: The percentage of employees who are employed in businesses that offer insurance
- Enrollment-when-eligible: The percentage of employees who meet the criteria for enrollment and actually enroll in employee-sponsored health insurance plans
- Enrollment: The percentage of all workers (eligible and non-eligible) who enroll in employee-sponsored health insurance plans offered to employees
- Eligibility: The percentage of employees who meet the criteria for eligibility to enroll

46. B: The primary determinant as to whether people enroll in employer-sponsored health coverage is the cost to the applicant. The higher the cost, the less likely employees are to enroll. For this reason, some companies offer a range of plans with different costs. Companies may make varying contributions to the cost of the insurance plans, ranging from 100% to 0%. Salary is another important consideration with those with higher salaries more likely to purchase insurance.

47. D: Resource utilization groups (RUGs) and minimum data sets (MDSs) are used to establish payment rates for skilled nursing facilities and help determine reimbursement under Medicare's PPS program. There are currently 53 RUGs with the RUG determined by the clients ADL score, use of therapy (based on minutes of therapy), services (intravenous therapy, respiratory therapy), functional ability, and medical conditions. The MDS is an assessment instrument used to evaluate service use and client characteristics.

48. C: A point of service plan is a structure that combines aspects of an HMO with a PPO. Clients are able to receive care from health care providers within the network or may seek treatment outside the network in some circumstances. This type of plan offers more flexibility to the client, but usually there are additional costs when a client chooses to seek treatment outside of the network. Copayments may increase and the percentage of costs covered by the plan may decrease.

49. B: The independent practice association (IPA) HMO model allows individual or groups of physicians to contract with an HMO to provide services while the physicians are also seeing non-HMO clients. The physicians maintain private practices and contract to serve clients enrolled in the HMO. In the staff model, physicians are hired by and work directly for the HMO. In the group practice model, the HMO has a contract with a large multi-specialty group that primarily sees HMO clients. With the direct contract model, the HMO contracts directly with a physician to provide services, and there is no insurer.

50. D: Health insurance is based on the principle of risk pooling. The insurance company enrolls large numbers of applicants, assuming that not all applicants will require payouts, so that the company can pay out benefits to only a portion of the applicants and still make a substantial profit. The law of large numbers is utilized to determine statistical probabilities related to mortality and morbidity in a specific time frame based on the pool of applicants.

51. C: A client who is temporarily disabled and has short-term disability insurance should usually expect to collect 60% of pre-disability salary after the client has used up all of the sick time. Short-term disability insurance usually covers a period of up to 6 months, although this may vary somewhat. However, clients must return to work when the disability is resolved, so many collect for only a brief period. Typical examples of short-term disabilities include pregnancy, back injuries, and fractures.

52. B: According to the American with Disabilities Act (ADA), public transportation must provide lifts that can accommodate occupied manual or powered wheelchairs that weigh up to 600 pounds. However, if the lift is able to support greater weight, the operator must accommodate those with weights greater than 600 pounds to the weight limit of the lift. The ADA also requires that the lifts accommodate wheelchairs up to 30 by 48 inches in width and length.

53. C: The government entity that requires that personal protective equipment be readily available at the worksite and in appropriate sizes is the Occupational Safety and Health Administration (OSHA). OSHA sets and enforces regulations related to workplace safety. In health care, this encompasses bloodborne pathogens, hazardous materials and hazardous wastes, and compressed gases and air equipment. OSHA also establishes lifting limits and ergonomic guidelines to minimize the risk of injury. Compliance officers can take complaints and issue citations for those out of compliance.

54. B: The FDA will allow emergency use of a drug with filing of an Investigational New Drug (IND) exemption for one client only and only one time per institution. The client's condition must be life-threatening or extremely debilitating and with no available standard treatment. There must be insufficient time to follow protocol to gain approval from the review committee, but a report must be filed with the review committee within 5 days. Consent must be obtained from the client or client's designee prior to administration of the drug.

55. D: Under Health Insurance Portability and Accountability Act (HIPAA) regulations, clients who request copies of laboratory results or other medical records must generally receive them within 30 days. A client or client designee may request laboratory results from the physician or directly from the laboratory. The request may have to be submitted in writing, and the client or client's designee may have to pay any costs, such as for CDs, copying, and mailing.

56. A: The CMS Clinical Quality Measures, in their Adult Recommended Core Measures, recommend that screening for depression (NQF 0418) begin at age 12. Other core measure includes controlling hypertension, avoiding high-risk medications in elderly patients, screening and cessation intervention for tobacco use, use of imaging for low back pain, documenting current medications, BMI screening and follow-up, receiving a specialist report, and completing functional status assessment.

57. A: Clients with a BMI outside of normal parameters should have a follow-up intervention plan in place and documented. The normal parameters for those who are 18 to 64 years of age are 18.5-25, so a BMI above 25 indicates the need for intervention. Normal BMI parameters for those age 65 and older are 23-30. BMI is based on height and weight, but clients should be assessed individually because muscle mass may affect results.

58. C: The best solution to dealing with a client who expresses extreme prejudice toward ethnic minorities and the LGBT population is to provide professional services and avoid debate. The case manager should stay focused on the needs of the client rather than the client's attitudes. Case managers often encounter ethical conflicts and clients with value systems at odds with their own, and trying to change the client's ideas is generally fruitless and just leads to conflict.

59. C: The Agency for Healthcare Research and Quality (AHRQ) provides clinical guidelines and recommendations. AHRQ maintains the National Guideline Clearinghouse (NGC), which is a database with evidence-based clinical practice guidelines. Health care professionals may submit guidelines to the NGC, which provides guidance in submission and inclusion criteria. AHRQ provides information to clients and consumers as well as health care professionals and policymakers. AHRQ also produces videos (available on YouTube through AHRQ Health TV) for clients and clinicians.

60. B: The primary purpose of a benchmark study is to compare an organization's performance against best practices of the industry to identify gaps in performance. Benchmark studies usually focus on specific processes or services and help to develop methods to adapt best practices to the workplace in order to improve performance. Benchmark studies may focus on clinical (such as outcomes of care), financial (such as cost-effectiveness, length of stay), or operational (such as the case management system in place) issues.

61. A: When conducting a client needs assessment as part of caseload calculations, the most important factors are:

- Acuity: Includes clinical characteristics. Increased clinical needs, such as with multiple morbidities or severe trauma, increased need for case manager time.
- Personal and family psychosocial issues: Issues may include cognitive impairment, psychological or mental illness, conflict, spiritual needs, ability of family/caregivers to assist in client care, needs of family and caregivers, and belief systems.
- Environment: Includes transitions of care.

62. D: The primary purpose of predictive modeling is to identify clients at risk for negative outcomes because of their clinical condition, health history, and various other factors (pharmacy utilization, health insurance claims) so that the case manager can take a proactive approach to intervention and prevention. Predictive modeling produces a Risk Index (RI) that helps to identify clients who can benefit from case management. Predictive modeling may be used in conjunction with other forms of assessment, such as assessing client acuity.

63. C: The purpose of a concurrent review (also known as continued stay review) of a hospitalized client is to assess the client's need for continued hospitalization as well as to assess the client's level of care. For example, a client may be assessed to determine if continued ICU care is necessary or if the client can be moved to a primary care unit. This type of review is done on an ongoing, often daily, basis during the client's hospitalization.

64. A: General Recovery is the Milliman Care Guideline that would be appropriate for clients with complex clinical situations and diagnoses for which a specific guideline does not exist. Chronic care provides guidelines for outpatient care for 20 chronic conditions. Inpatient and surgical care provides guidelines for clients needing hospitalization and/or surgery. Ambulatory care provides guidelines for managing outpatient referrals, diagnostic procedures, rehabilitation services, and pharmaceutical utilization. Home care provides guidelines for home health care, and recovery facility care provides guidelines for admission to recovery facilities and discharge planning.

65. A: Focused utilization management programs that target only specific client populations often result in cost savings and improved care. Cost savings are derived from limiting the scope of utilization management so it requires fewer staff hours as well as from better provision of care resulting from the process. Utilization management, for example, may focus on high-risk clients or chronic care client, areas in which early intervention and appropriate referrals and coordination of care have the potential to improve client outcomes.

66. C: Under the hospice benefit for end-of-life care, *home* is defined as any place the client is residing, and this can include jail, residential care facilities, primary residences, or licensed health care facilities. The aim of hospice care is to provide comfort care in the "home" environment with support for not only the client but also family members and caregivers. Hospice provides services needed to maintain the client in the home, including home health aide, social services, durable medical equipment, pain medication, and medical supplies.

67. A: Core indicators of end-stage disease are those that are common among a wide range of clients, regardless of diagnosis. Core indicators include serum albumin less than 2.5 g/dL, decline in physical condition, presence of multiple morbidities, assistance needed for most ADLs, Karnofsky score 50% or less, and the client expressing a desire to die. In addition to core indicators, there are disease-specific indicators. For example, stroke clients often exhibit decreased level of consciousness, dysphagia, dementia, and increased medical complications.

68. D: Domain is the term that refers to a case manager's area of practice and sphere of knowledge. Function comprises the actions that the case manager carries out in fulfilling the job requirements. Role refers to the function, job title, or position of the case manager. Venue (also referred to as context) refers to the specific type of organization or institution for which the case manager is employed and the type of population the case manager serves.

69. C: A Karnofsky Performance Status Scale score of 30 indicates that the client is severely disabled and unable to attend to ADLs independently and likely requires institutional or hospital care. The Karnofsky Performance Status Scale classifies clients according to their functional abilities and impairments with scores ranging from 100 (normal with no indications of disease) to 0 (death). Score of 80 to 100 indicate the client is independent in care, 50 to 70 indicates the inability to work but the ability to live at home with some assistance at times. Scores of 10 to 40 indicate the need for institutionalization/hospitalization.

70. B: A client's case management plan should focus on establishing goals and prioritizing needs. The plan is developed from the results on a client assessment. Establishing goals includes identification of strategies for care and interventions and considers the need for resources. While the need for cost-effective care is always important, it should not be the primary focus of the case management plan. The plan should be multidisciplinary and should decrease the risk of negative outcomes.

71. A: A discharge planning evaluation must include an evaluation of the client's need for post-hospitalization services and the availability of those services. The client must also be evaluated for the ability to manage self-care and to be cared for within the environment from which the client was initially admitted. Clients should be assessed on admission to determine the need for discharge planning. These clients should include all those at risk for adverse effects after discharge in the absence of discharge planning.

72. D: The purpose of admission certification is to determine the medical necessity of admission to a hospital or other health care institution. Admission certification is a form of utilization management that is carried out prior to admission to ensure clients will get the appropriate level of care and usually includes estimates of length of stay for the client's diagnosis. Admission certification is not a determination of benefits, so it does not guarantee care will be paid for.

73. B: The case manager should always avoid dual relationships with clients. While it is unethical to have a sexual or romantic relationship with a client, serious problems can also arise if the case manager has other relationships with a client. The case manager should not work with neighbors, friends, relatives, or other acquaintances because the case manager is in the position of power, making decisions about the client's care; this may result in perceptions of abuse of power or conflict of interest.

74. D: The case manager should give out no information about the client and should not even acknowledge the client is at the hospital because this is a violation of the patient's right to confidentiality unless the client has given permission for his wife to receive information and a method of accurate identification, such as a password, is set up in advance. Anyone can telephone and pose as a family member to get information, so the case manager must use great care.

75. B: The case manager may break a client's confidentiality only under limited circumstances, which include when a client is in need of emergent care and this care necessitates information (for example, if a client has taken an overdose of a particular drug). Other circumstances include when clients pose a risk of harm to themselves or others. Confidentiality may be breached when discussing the client's condition with a supervisor. Clients may be referred to collection services if they fail to pay for services in a reasonable time frame.

76. D: An appropriate statement for a case manager to make on a social networking site about working with clients is no statement whatsoever! The case manager should not describe clients, even in general terms without naming them, because people may be able to determine whom the case manager refers by the description. Additionally, complaining about work ("I have to see way too many clients") suggests that the case manager is not able to give adequate attention to clients.

77. A: The best tool to combat fear of technology and data is education. Since much of medical care is now data driven, the case manager must deal with data on a daily basis, and staff members must become used to an evidence-based focus on providing care. Staff members may require technical computer training in order to use electronic records more effectively and should become familiar with the types of data that are collected and analyzed.

78. C: To increase compliance, the case manager who institutes changes in procedures in order to improve patient outcomes should include accountability. For example, a procedure may require that a checklist be completed and documented. Initially, the changes should be communicated and explained to staff, but this alone does not always bring about compliance because staff members often resort to familiar procedures, especially if they are busy and less familiar with the new procedure.

79. D: The factor that has the most significant effect on hospital length of stay is the client's diagnosis, accounting for over 25% of variations in length of stay. Length of stay also increases with comorbidities and with the number of surgical procedures. Age is another important factor, as elderly patients tend to have longer hospital stays than younger clients, although this is an additive factor superimposed upon diagnosis. Clients who receive discharge planning early in their hospital stay tend to have shorter lengths of stay than clients who receive later discharge planning.

80. A: When the client of a mental health case manager refuses case management after being discharged from a mental institution, the case manager should assess the need for court-ordered case management by determining if the client appears to pose a threat to self or others. The case manager must consider the patient's history, diagnosis, and circumstances of admission to the facility and discharge, as well as the client's compliance with treatment and potential for growth.

81. B: When doing financial analysis of diagnosis-related groups (DRGs), *relative weights* refers to value assigned to DRG based on complexity and resources needed. Complexity usually refers to the number of different services required for treatment. Some diagnoses may fall within only one DRG while other diagnoses may fall within a number of DRGs, all with different relative weights assigned. When relative weights are high, reimbursement increases, so some institutions may favor admissions with high relative weights.

82. D: When doing case management evaluation using the cost-effectiveness analysis method, *sensitivity analysis* refers to testing assumptions and validating conclusions in order to determine if there are alternate explanations that could explain costs and benefits. The cost-effectiveness analysis method includes 6 principles: (1) statement of analytic perspective, (2) description of anticipated benefits, (3) outline of types of costs, (4) adjustment for differential timing (discounting), (5) sensitivity analysis, and (6) summary of measurement of efficiency (cost-effectiveness ratio).

83. A: While regulations vary somewhat from state to state, generally assisted living facilities must have 24-hour staffing to assist clients with ADLs, housekeeping, recreation, transportation, and medication management, but skilled nursing care is not required. Different types of assisted living facilities include group homes, adult foster care, residential care facilities, and sheltered housing. Assisted living facilities or care may be provided in continuing-care communities in which clients may first live independently, before they move to an area that provides assisted care as the need arises.

84. D: The best placement for a 24-year-old client with schizophrenia being discharged from a psychiatric institution for the first time in 4 years is likely a group home that specializes in clients with mental illness and provides medication monitoring and assistance with community services and managing budget, cooking, and housekeeping. Clients who have spent prolonged periods in psychiatric facilities may need to spend 6 to 12 months in a group home before transitioning into less supervised living situations.

85. B: The average length of stay in an acute hospital for a client at least 65 years of age with septicemia ranges from approximately 8 to 10 days, depending on the age and gender, with those older than 85 years having slightly shorter lengths of stay than those younger than 85. Average length of stay is determined by dividing the days of acute care by the number of discharges based on a sampling of clients with diagnoses based on the International Classification of Disease.

86. D: An emergent group is one that emerges as a result of mutual interest over time, and can include a group of friends. In a work environment, this type of emergent group usually does not have specific goals, unlike planned groups, but can influence attitudes. Emergent groups do not have explicit rules but an unstated understanding of the behavior that is consistent with the group norm. The group boundaries tend to be more fluid than in planned groups, so members may come and go.

87. C: A case manager who influences members of a group but is not in turn influenced by the members is exemplifying unilateral interdependence. Interdependence occurs when people's attitudes, experiences, and feelings are influenced by someone else. With unilateral interdependence, the leader influences the followers but the lack of mutual influence suggests an autocratic relationship, which may be useful in emergent situations but may impair group dynamics as followers feel they have no voice.

88. A: In dealing with conflict, a staff person who follows the guidelines of the case manager he or she disagrees with is exhibiting accommodation, which is cooperative but nonassertive. Other modes of dealing with conflict include competing, collaborating, compromising, and avoiding. Competing and collaborating are assertive while avoiding and accommodating are unassertive behaviors. Avoiding and competing are uncooperative while collaborating and accommodating are cooperative. Compromising is the middle ground between asserting and cooperating and between competing and accommodating.

89. C: When evaluating research, the P value that is most statistically significant is 0.002. The P value estimates the probability that the null hypothesis will be rejected. For example, if comparing two treatments, the null hypothesis states there is no difference in outcomes, so rejecting the null hypothesis means that a difference exists. If the P value is <0.05, this difference is generally considered to be statistically significant. A P value of 0.002 would be highly significant.

90. A: When conducting an interview, the case manager should avoid questions that begin with "why" because they require the person being interviewed to provide a reason. Not only do some people find it difficult to explain their actions, but they also may simply feel providing reasons is an invasion of their privacy and intrusive. "Why" questions can also seem accusatory to some people, as if the case manager is finding fault with their actions or choices.

91. B: "Sentinel procedures" refers to those procedures (often diagnostic) associated with life-threatening diseases or conditions. When clients are undergoing sentinel procedures, this should alert the case manager for the potential need for case management services even if the initial diagnoses do not indicate a need, as the ultimate diagnosis may be far more life-threatening. Sentinel procedures includes exploratory laparotomy, organ (heart, lung, liver, kidney, brain, bone marrow) and lymph node biopsies, and insertion of arteriovenous shunt.

92. C: When making decisions about case management based on catastrophic diagnoses, diagnoses would include solid-organ transplants because the potential for costly and time-consuming complications is very high. These clients often have very high rates of utilization of resources because of the need for multiple health care providers and procedures. Other catastrophic diagnoses include HIV/AIDS, kidney failure, liver failure, traumatic brain injuries, cancer/leukemia, acute respiratory distress syndrome, respiratory distress syndrome of infancy, premature delivery, and multi-trauma cases. Patients undergoing neurological surgery also may have multiple complications.

93. D: Passive acquisition of cases refers to acquisition by referral from health care providers, such as from physicians or nursing staff who determine a client is in need of case management, often based on a change in the client's diagnosis or condition that results in increased need for services. This type of acquisition of clients is becoming more common as health care providers become more familiar with the services the case manager provides, especially when the case manager is an active member of a team.

94. A: The best response to a client who is progressing well after a stroke (or any illness/injury) but remains extremely fearful and anxious about discharge is to explore the client's concerns with the client, allowing the client to express his or her feelings. The person may have valid reasons for concerns, such as living alone or lack of transportation, and may not fully understand the services that are available in the community or may feel overwhelmed by changes in physical condition and abilities.

95. C: The best method of sharing data with staff about the positive outcomes of case management is by providing charts and graphs because they are easy to interpret and information can be gleaned very quickly. Percentages are the weakest of all statistics because they can be easily manipulated. Raw data are hard to interpret, as they require the viewer to make conclusions and sometimes do calculations. Narrative explanations are more time-consuming to the viewer and may be a useful addition to charts and graphs rather than as stand-alone presentation of data.

96. B: When preparing a quality improvement report, the case manager should begin by identifying the indicator that was measured (such as length of stay for myocardial infarction), providing any necessary background information or historical statistics. Then, the case manager should outline interventions utilized to bring about improvement. The case manager should explain the type of measurement used for assessment and the final results of that assessment. The results may be presented in various formats, but visual formats (charts, graphs) are usually the easiest for staff to interpret.

97. B: When completing a cost-benefit analysis, an example of a "soft" cost savings is prevention of complications. Soft cost savings refer to those costs that are avoided and are difficult to calculate directly based on one patient, but may be calculated over time by looking at multiple patients and historical costs. "Hard" savings are those that relate directly to actions taken by the case manager, such as decreased length of hospitalization stay, client's change to a provider in the network, and transfer from an acute level of care to a lower level of care.

98. A: The case manager who wants to justify further intervention for a rehabilitation client who has not met performance goals should begin with the data on admission to the program. For example, if one of the goals is the ability to walk up 2 flights of stairs, the beginning data may include the ability to walk up and down 3 steps. This should be followed by the current data, such as the ability to walk up one flight of stairs. Then, the case manager should outline the goal and any pertinent information.

99. D: A client who refuses to talk to the case manager because her husband had a bad experience with a case manager is exhibiting a barrier to communication involving perceptions. The client has a preconceived negative impression of the case manager and the case manager services based on her husband's experience, even though it may be totally unrelated. The case manager should acknowledge the problems the husband encountered and encourage the client to express her feelings openly to begin to build a relationship of trust.

100. A: Prior to the initial interview with a client, the case manager should review the client's medical records, including both current records and records of previous hospitalization or care. The case manager should make an appointment and tell the client whom the case manager represents (hospital, insurance company) and how long the appointment should take. The case manager should introduce himself/herself to the client and take time to establish rapport with the client before beginning the formal interview and assessment. The case manager should summarize findings and discuss the plan of care at the end of the interview.

101. C: While all of these are important considerations for the client with multiple comorbidities and multiple physicians, these clients are especially at risk for polypharmacy so one of the first assessments should be medication reconciliation. This should be done initially and after any intervention, such as a visit to the physician or a hospitalization. The case manager should assess the medications, the prescribing physicians, the client's knowledge about the medications, and the client's method, dosage, and frequency of taking the medications; clients often fail to take medications as prescribed.

102. D: The focus of case management in a pre-acute environment, such as a physician's office or clinic, is often on prevention, reducing the need for costly medical interventions and hospitalization. This may include monitoring client's medications and treatments to ensure compliance, doing assessment of health risks, facilitating health screenings, as well as encouraging lifestyle changes, such as increased exercise and smoking cessation, and enrolling clients in wellness programs. The case manager may do telephone triage and monitoring and make referrals to community agencies to provide the client necessary resources.

103. B: In negotiating prices with an out-of-network health care provider or any other negotiating, the case manager should begin by researching prices and coming to the negotiation well prepared. Negotiations may be aggressive, with one side perceived as a winner and the other side as a loser, but this type of negotiation often impairs relationships and may negatively impact future negotiations. Negotiations may also be cooperative, with each side working together to find a mutually satisfying solution. Cooperative negotiations are usually more productive and establish better working relationships.

104. A: The primary goal of quality improvement projects is to evaluate where and how medical errors occur rather than to assign blame. Reducing errors often serves to increase cost savings. Errors may include failure to provide adequate care and inefficient procedures, as well as direct errors, such as giving the wrong medication. Objectives include reducing the overall medical errors and associated morbidities and mortality, developing best practices, improving client satisfaction with care, promoting safety, and improving professional performance of duties.

105. C: The clinical resources model is the model of acute care case management that follows the client's progress through acute hospitalization to ensure effective, safe, and cost-effective transition from acute care to post-acute care. The integrated functional model refers to case management that includes the responsibility for both utilization review and discharge planning. The disease management model focuses on post-acute care for chronic diseases in order to reduce rehospitalization. The outcomes management model focuses on improving clinical outcomes and cost-effectiveness in the acute care environment.

106. D: In a payer-based case management model, the case manager is generally an employee of the insurance company and must ensure that the client receives competent and quality care while still ensuring that the care is cost-effective. Payer-based case management may present the case manager with ethical dilemmas because the insurance company may be more focused on cost-effectiveness than client needs; however, the case manager must retain the role of client advocate and try to balance concerns.

107. A: The most common reasons for screening clients to determine need for case management are diagnosis, high rates of resource utilization (often exemplified by repeat or frequent hospitalizations and visits to emergency department), and high costs of care in dollar amounts (usually within a set duration of time, such as the preceding 6 to 12 months). This type of screening is often automated so that these clients are tagged on admission and referred to case management. This may exclude some clients whose diagnosis and/or condition changes after admission.

108. C: Physical disability: Defect in body function, such as may occur with chronic conditions, such as osteoarthritis in the knees. Sensory disability: Vision and hearing deficits as well as impaired sense of taste and smell, touch, and balance. Intellectual disability: Cognitive impairment (intellectual disability, dementia). Mental disability: Mental health disorder that impairs functioning. Pervasive developmental disability: Impaired ability to socialize and communicate, such as with autism. Developmental disability: Impaired growth and development, such as with spina bifida.

109. B: The Chronic Care Model is primarily utilized in the primary care setting and focuses on providing case management to those with chronic illnesses in order to improve client outcomes through prevention. Clients are considered active participants in their own care. The components of the model include the health system that is involved, the delivery system of care (team members and roles), the use of evidence-based guidelines for decision support and integrated care of primary physician and specialists, clinical information systems, and utilization of community resources.

110. D: In the Patient-Centered Medical Home Model of care, the team leader coordinating care is usually the client's personal physician with whom the client has an ongoing relationship; the physician understands the needs of the client and can lead the team in providing the resources the client needs throughout the patient's life stages and continuum of care. The physician serves as a patient advocate and utilizes evidence-based practices and clinical decision support tools and information technology as well as continuous quality improvement. Clients are active participants in care.

111. C: Palliative care is intended for those who need to improve their quality of life by managing symptoms. Palliative care can begin at any point during an illness and is unrelated to diagnosis or life expectancy. Unlike hospice care, palliative care clients can be undergoing curative treatments. Many clients with life-threatening diseases or chronic illnesses may begin with palliative care for control of pain or other symptoms and then may progress to hospice care as their condition deteriorates and they opt to have no further curative treatments.

112. B: Clients who are receiving physical therapy as part of community rehabilitation through a home health agency can expect to receive 30 minutes to 1 hour of therapy, usually 3 days a week per therapist. If the client is receiving therapy from multiple therapists (physical therapist, occupational therapist, speech therapist), then this time limit applies to each therapist. Under original Medicare, an episode of care comprises 60 days. In order to avoid extra costs, the client should receive therapy from a home health agency that is Medicare certified.

113. A: The case manager realizes that when a client transitions between providers, the client is at increased risk for complication and negative outcomes because the new provider (whether in a different level of care or in a different facility) may have insufficient knowledge of the client's condition and history. Inadequate communication may result in incorrect treatments, medication errors, and neglect of client needs. New providers may not be clear about who is responsible for different aspects of care, so the case manager must ensure continuity of care.

114. D: Standards of practice include statements that outline the level of performance expected of a professional, such as a case manager. The standards of practice are usually developed by professional organizations, especially those that provide certification. Case management plans outline client care procedures and expected outcomes. Standards of care outline the level of care that all clients should expect, based on evidence-based practice and outcomes data. Evidence-based practice guidelines outline care that should be provided for specific diagnoses/conditions.

115. B: In an acute hospital interdisciplinary team, the individual primarily responsible for assessing the post-discharge needs of the client is the case manager. While all members of the team collaborate to provide care within the acute hospital and some may be actively involved in planning for post-discharge needs, the responsibility still remains with the case manager who must not only identify needs but determine the community resources available to meet those needs and make arrangements for necessary community providers.

116. A: In order to qualify for inpatient rehabilitation, a client must be able to undergo rehabilitation therapy for at least 3 hours daily for 5 to 7 days per week. If clients require therapy but cannot tolerate this many hours of therapy, then they may be transferred to a skilled nursing facility, which requires that the clients need skilled care daily (including rehabilitation therapy and/or medical treatments) and are medically stable. Sub-acute care is available for clients who do not still require acute care but require more care than is available in a skilled nursing facility.

117. C: A swing bed agreement with CMS allows a hospital to use the same bed for acute or skilled nursing facility (SNF) care, depending on the needs of the client. This agreement is used primarily for small or rural facilities where alternate types of facilities offering different levels of care are not readily available in the community. Clients may be admitted into acute care and transitioned to SNF care while staying in the same room and bed, although the level of care that they receive will be different.

118. D: Most medical insurance will not cover intermediate care, which is a level of care slightly more intense than custodial care. The client may require nursing supervision but does not require skilled medical care or therapy. Medical insurance also does not generally cover custodial care, although in some instances Medicaid does provide custodial care. Custodial care provides clients assistance with activities of daily living and may also include homemaking services, such as cooking and cleaning.

119. B: The purpose of health coaching (also referred to as wellness coaching) is to help clients achieve their goals. The case manager encourages the client to identify their own problems and set goals for change, serving as a support rather than an instructor. The primary role of the case manager is to listen and respond. The case manager helps the clients explore ways of achieving their goals and monitors their progress as they make positive changes.

120. D: The Rancho Los Amigos Levels of Cognitive Functioning tool is used to evaluate traumatic brain injuries. According to the tool, a client with a score of VIII is exhibiting appropriate behavior. The scale runs from I to VIII with I at one end of the scale indicating unresponsiveness to all types of stimuli and VIII at the other end of the scale (purposeful, appropriate response). A revised scale (I to X) is also used in some places and includes descriptions of ability to function (needs assistance, independent).

121. A: The most useful way in which to divide groups of clients is by risk stratification. Once the case manager has established groups of clients in similar situations, then the groups are divided by risk stratification (usually through a software program) into those at low risk, medium risk, and high risk so that the case manager can focus efforts on those with the greatest need. In any large group of clients, usually about 20% are at high risk and will need more resources.

122. C: If a $100,000 investment in hiring a case manager results in savings of $120,000, then $20,000 represents the return on investment (ROI). With ROI, the returns may be in the form of profit or savings, although savings may be more difficult to calculate with accuracy. ROI is calculated for a specific period of time, usually 1 year.

123. A: Disease management programs are usually intended for specific populations of clients, usually those identified as at high risk because of diagnosis, complications, and history of resource utilization and high costs. Part of planning the program is to research data and identify barriers to change before implementing interventions. Often pilot programs and/or focus groups are utilized to evaluate interventions. The implemented program usually includes the use of clinical practice guidelines to promote consistency and a process to evaluate outcomes.

124. B: The case manager working with clients with substance abuse usually focuses on assisting clients to obtain needed resources. Care for those with substance abuse is often fragmented and may be costly, so the case manager must be aware of all resources in the community, such as outpatient treatment centers and 12-step programs. Clients with substance abuse often have dual diagnoses and may need treatment for mental or medical health problems as well as substance abuse. Some may be homeless and may need information about shelters and meal programs.

125. C: When a client tells the case manager that her caregiver does not allow her to use the telephone or read her mail, the case manager should suspect that the client is experiencing psychological abuse. Psychological abuse may include threats, coercion, and intimidation, as well as behavior that is controlling (and often isolating), such as preventing a client access to mail or the telephone. Nurses are mandatory reporters of abuse, so any evidence of abuse should be reported to the proper authorities.

126. B: A client who is a devoutly religious Catholic and believes her health problems are punishment for sins may benefit most from pastoral counseling because a priest who is trained as a therapist may help the client balance religious and health beliefs in a more realistic manner. Pastoral counselors often carry out both psychological and spiritual counseling, providing the client with the support of the faith community. Pastoral counselors may represent many different faiths and branches of religions.

127. C: When doing telephonic case management, the primary focus is usually on triaging clients to determine which clients have emergent needs requiring immediate attention, urgent needs and can be referred to a primary care physician with 8 to 24 hours, and non-urgent needs and can provide self-care with guidance from the case manager. Case managers are commonly used in managed care organizations in order to prevent negative health outcomes and hospitalization, utilize resources wisely, and reduce costs.

128. D: A warning sign that a case manager is developing a relationship with a client that is too personal is the case manager asking the client about personal matters unrelated to the client's needs. It's common to enjoy interacting with some clients more than others or even feel some attraction to a client, but the case manager should recognize signs and avoid acting on any attraction or showing preference for one client over others, while maintaining a professional relationship at all times.

129. C: When a client has signed a release of information form so the case manager can provide information to a therapist or any other individual, the case manager should release the minimum information necessary to meet the request. If for example, the request does not include the initial assessment or progress notes, then the case manager should not include those with the records released. Even when records are released, the case manager should remain aware of the client's right to confidentiality and privacy.

130. C: A terminally ill client who believes that prayer will heal her probably depends on faith for comfort. A deeply held belief in the power of prayer is common to many who are profoundly religious and does not mean the client is in denial or not dealing realistically with his or her condition. For example, Christian Scientists routinely turn to prayer to heal sickness and eschew medicine, and believe that it is God's will if they are not healed.

131. A: A bipolar client who is very nervous about transitioning into the community from a sheltered environment may benefit from a support group comprised of people dealing with similar issues. Support groups may have a mental health professional as a leader. Support groups are usually open groups that allow clients to choose whether or not to attend, but the groups provide a safe and supportive atmosphere where people can discuss shared concerns and methods of coping.

132. B: According to the Transtheoretical Model of change, the process of change that people go through when they express feelings (positive and negative) about change is dramatic relief. People go through 5 stages when attempting to change: precontemplation, contemplation, preparation, action, and maintenance. People also go through 10 processes at each stage of change. Processes include consciousness raising, counterconditioning, dramatic relief, environmental reevaluation, helping relationships, reinforcement management, self-liberation, self-evaluation, social liberation, and stimulus control.

133. A: In Robert's Seven-Stage Crisis Intervention Model, the first stage includes assessing lethality and the potential for danger. Seven stages include:

1. Psychosocial/Lethality assessment
2. Rapid establishment of rapport by showing respect, making eye contact, and being positive
3. Identify major problems/precipitants and prioritize, discussing client's current coping mechanisms
4. Deal with feelings/emotions, encouraging client to vent and using therapeutic communication
5. Generate and explore alternatives, collaboratively with client
6. Implement plan of action
7. Follow-up/Evaluation

134. D: Clients with schizophrenia, depression, or bipolar disease are at high risk for dual diagnosis as many clients self-medicate with alcohol or illicit drugs. These clients often need enrollment in a program that targets both problems, as the approach to treatment for substance abuse is different for mentally ill clients than for those who are not mentally ill. Programs for dual diagnosis clients tend to be more supportive and less confrontational. Peer support is also important to treatment.

135. D: The Digit Repetition Test is primarily used to diagnose attention deficits in those with normal intelligence. The test requires the client to listen and repeat numbers, starting with two random single-digit numbers (such as 3,7) and then adding a third number to a different sequence (such as 7,4,9) each time the client answers correctly. A normal score for a person with average intelligence is the ability to repeat 5 to 7 numbers. A score below 5 indicates impaired attention.

136. D: A client who insists that the case manager sit down with the client and explain the health care options in detail and outline them in writing is exhibiting self-advocacy by insisting on what he or she needs to understand and make decisions. Self-advocacy involves a client speaking up and becoming an active participant in planning and making decisions about care. Clients who advocate for themselves are more likely to want to be involved in self-care and to remain in compliance with treatment.

137. A: An elderly low-income home care client who is losing weight because she doesn't like to cook and lives on junk food may benefit most from meal delivery services, as her diet is the immediate problem. Home meal delivery services (such as Meals on Wheels) are usually reasonably priced and provide food for one to three meals daily, depending on the specific program. Assisted living facilities and homemaker services may be too expensive for a low-income client and are not usually covered by Medicare or insurance companies.

138. D: If an uninsured client who is ineligible for Medicaid is unable to pay for an expensive chemotherapeutic drug, the initial step in solving the problem is to determine if the drug company has a pharmaceutical assistance program. Most drug companies have such programs, usually intended for those who are uninsured or underinsured and meet specific criteria for need. Some programs are drug-specific. Some states also have pharmaceutical assistance programs, especially for AIDS drugs.

139. B: RotaCare clinics are supported by health care volunteers and Rotary Clubs and provide free medical care to the uninsured, underinsured, and homeless. The clinics are located throughout the United States and treat clients with minor illnesses and injuries. Some clinics also have specialty clinics with a range of different specialists, such as dermatologists or psychiatrists, while others have lists of physicians and dentists willing to provide *pro bono* care for clients. Some clinics provide vaccinations and HIV testing as well as wellness programs and health education.

140. A: The case manager who cannot find food or shelter for a homeless client may receive assistance for the client from the local Salvation Army, which is a Christian denominational church with international charities. While programs vary from city to city, the Salvation Army usually has programs for the homeless in most areas and often provides meals and shelter or emergency funds. The Salvation runs a network of thrift stores to support rehabilitation programs for substance abuse.

141. B: A client who suffers from posttraumatic stress syndrome, which interferes with his ability to work and communicate with others, would be best classified as having a psychiatric disability because the client's condition interferes with his ability to function. Although some patients stabilize and go into remission with medication and treatment, because of the erratic nature of much mental illness, many clients have a psychiatric disability and may be eligible for Social Security disability payments.

142. C: While grief responses vary widely and the length of bereavement varies as well, because the client is having much difficulty functioning and caring for her home and family, her grieving process is exaggerated, so she will probably benefit most from referral to a bereavement counselor who can help the client move toward a more normal grieving process. As part of counselling, the counselor may suggest that the client participate in a support group for people whose spouses have died.

143. D: Self-directed Medicaid services allow participants to make decisions over certain specified services. The participant may use Medicaid funds to hire a personal aide or an individual person to provide care that would otherwise be done by the client or a skilled provider. For example, a client no longer able to do intermittent catheterization may be allowed to hire, train, and supervise an individual person or personal aide to do this procedure. Self-directed Medicaid services may include both "employer authority" (hiring, training, supervising) and "budget authority" (determining how funds are distributed).

144. A: Depression is common in older adults with comorbid conditions and chronic conditions affecting the quality of life, such as cancer, diabetes, arthritis, and heart disease, with approximately 37% experiencing depression. Some medications, such as steroids, diuretics, and Parkinson disease drugs may also precipitate depression. Depression is often undiagnosed because screening for depression in older adults is often neglected. The Geriatric Depression Scale is a self-assessment tool that can be used to identify those with depression.

145. D: The instrument that is most appropriate to assess general health and disability across all medical disciplines, including mental, neurological, and substance abuse, is World Health Organization Disability Assessment Schedule 2 (WHODAS-2), which should now be used in place of the Global Assessment of Functioning (GAF) test. WHODAS-2 has 12-item and 36-item versions as well as self-administered and interviewer-administered versions. Domains include understanding and communicating, getting around, self-care, getting along with people, life activities, and participation in society.

146. C: A series of steps in treatment based on client response and developed through scientific- and evidence-based research in order to standardize a specific type of care is referred to as an algorithm. For example, Algorithms are widely used in emergency departments to determine treatment related to advanced cardiac life support. Algorithms may incorporate a decision-tree approach to aid in choosing the correct treatment. Some states (such as Texas) are using algorithms to advise Medicaid physicians about prescribing medications, such as antipsychotics.

147. B: The purpose of the Patient Activation Measure (PAM) is to assess the client's ability for self-care by evaluating knowledge about medications and condition and confidence in managing care. This instrument assesses 13 items with scores ranging from 0 (low ability) to 52 (high ability). Clients are placed into one of four levels of self-care based on their scores:

- Level 1: Client's role is passive.
- Level 2: Client lacks confidence in abilities and adequate understanding of health.
- Level 3: Client is beginning to build understanding, but still may lack confidence.
- Level 4: Client is managing self-care, but may falter with stress or health problems.

148. C: Adherence to the plan of care is important if the goals of case management are to be met, but there may be many barriers to adherence (lack of income, need to work, lack of assistance, pain), so the best solution to lack of adherence is to sit down with the client and, in a nonjudgmental manner, discuss the client's goals and any barriers the client has encountered in order to determine what steps can be taken to improve adherence.

149. A: When a client's condition does not progress according to expectations as outlined in the clinical pathway, this is referred to as a variance. For tracking purposes, when a variance occurs, it is classified according to where the cause lies—with the client, the physician, the nursing staff, other health care providers, or the system. A variance may result in a new pathway or an adjusted pathway, depending on the type of variance. In some cases, more than one pathway will be followed at the same time.

150. A: Force field analysis is a decision-making technique that comprises both consideration of restraining forces, which negatively impact a program, and driving forces, which positively impact the program. Restraining forces can include satisfaction with the status quo (or fear of change), lack of support from administration, lack of adequate resources, inadequate numbers of staff, lack of time, lack of knowledge, and fear of statistics. Driving forces can include the need or desire to predict needed skill sets, track present and future costs, improve outcomes, and remain current.

151. B: If an insurance company has denied coverage for therapy that the case manager feels should have been covered for a client, the first thing the case manager should do is assist the client to file an appeal. It is not unusual for insurance companies to deny coverage, and each company has an appeal process that should be followed. The letter of denial should provide the reason for denial, but if not, the client or client's representative should call to find out the reason so that it can be addressed in the appeal.

152. D: If a client was seriously injured at work but feel that the employer was negligent and plans to sue, the client should file suit and avoid applying for Workers' Compensation because Workers' Compensation regulations require that the individual that receives benefits relinquish the right to sue for negligence. Workers' Compensation is a state-run program that may vary somewhat from one state to another but is an insurance policy to cover wages and medical care for those injured at work.

153. C: A TRICARE beneficiary is eligible for TRICARE for Life if the person has both Medicare A and B. TRICARE for Life is a Medicare wrap-around program that allows clients to seek medical care from any Medicare provider, non-Medicare provider, military hospital, or clinic (if space is available). Claims are first paid for through Medicare and then forwarded to other healthcare

48

provider (if available) and then to TRICARE, which will pay the balance for TRICARE-covered services.

154. D: The billing code that is utilized for services such as ambulance and durable medical equipment is HCPCS-Level II. HCPCS codes are used for non-physician services. Codes comprise a letter (A, B, C, D...), which designates the category (such as E code: Durable Medical Equipment) followed by 4 numbers, which designate the specific item (such as E1130 to E1161 for different types of wheelchairs).

155. D: If the case manager wants to apply the correct diagnostic code for outpatient services to a billing form, the case manager would utilize ICD-10-CM. ICD-10 is used for diagnoses for both inpatient and outpatient services and is consistent with DSM-V, cancer registry codes, and nursing classifications. ICD-10-PCS contains procedure codes for inpatient procedures while CPT contains codes for outpatient procedures. HCPCS-Level II codes are utilized for durable medical equipment and other services, such as ambulance, not covered by other codes. NDC is national drug codes.

156. A: The term that would most apply to a transgender female (biological male) who is attracted to females is lesbian. While gay might also fit, this term is more commonly used to refer to male homosexuals. For legal and descriptive purposes, a transgender female is considered the same as a biological female when considering issues such as sexual attraction. Thus, a transgender male (biological female) who is attracted to females is considered heterosexual.

157. B: A case manager assigned to a population health program (which is geared toward improving the health of a particular group) in an African American community with high rates of hypertension and diabetes should initially focus education on diet and exercise because these lifestyle changes may be most effective in helping to manage both hypertension and diabetes. Interventions may include cooking and nutrition classes, support groups (especially for weight loss and diabetes), visits to farmers' markets, walking groups, and other types of exercise.

158. C: The case manager is preparing a client to undergo a functional capacity evaluation required by the client's insurance company following injury and tells the client that the evaluation will not include motivation. The FCE focuses on the ability of the client to carry out job functions and may include lifting ability, range of motion, stamina, strength measures, ability to carry items, and other physical activities that may be required by the specific type of job.

159. B: If a client with a disability is applying for a job and asks the case manager if he should disclose the disability to the employer, the best response is, "You only need to disclose if you expect an accommodation." If no accommodation is needed for the client to carry out job functions, then there is no legal requirement under the American with Disabilities Act for the client to disclose the information, and it is not legal for the employer to ask if an applicant has a disability. However, if informed about the disability, the employer can ask what accommodations, if any, are needed.

160. D: If the organization is using the John Hopkins ACG® (Adjusted Clinical Group) system, the case manager expects that it will help to predict clients' future health needs. This system considers all of the client's morbidity and healthcare history and experiences rather than the practice pattern of the clinician when assessing risk. The ACG system helps to better identify those clients who are at risk for further health problems and may benefit from case management and interventions.

161. A: When determining if a client has achieved a healthcare goal, such as lowered blood pressure, the case manager should observe and measure personally. While discussing outcomes with clients and reviewing records are important, the case manager should verify whenever possible because the case manager can then be sure that a goal was achieved. Additionally, if the case manager is engaged in monitoring, the client is more likely to try to comply with treatment and work toward achieving goals.

162. C: If the case manager is concerned that a client's attention seems to wonder, the best test to assess attention is the Digit Repetition Test. The client is asked to listen to numbers and then repeat them. The case manager starts with two random single-digit numbers. If the client gets this sequence correct, the case manager then states 3 numbers and continues to add one number each time until the client is unable to repeat the numbers correctly. People with normal intelligence (without retardation or expressive aphasia) can usually repeat 5 to 7 numbers, so scores < 5 indicate impaired attention.

163. B: If a client with COPD has tried repeatedly to quit smoking but feels that quitting is impossible, the case manager should provide support and assist the client in establishing short and long-term goals. For some clients who are very resistive to quitting, cutting back on smoking may be an initial goal, and the case manager may suggest chewing nicotine gum, sucking on hard candy, or other activity when the client feels the urge to smoke.

164. D: While all of these are important, the primary reason for stratifying risk is to provide preventive intervention before problems arise. During risk stratification, clients who are at high risk of incurring rehospitalizations or increased medical costs are identified and intervention plans made to ensure that the client has adequate follow up and treatment in order to reduce utilization of health care services. Clients are placed into high-risk, moderate risk, or low risk categories.

165. A: If the case manager contacts the pharmacist regarding a client's medications and verified the prescriptions with the physician, this meets the case management goal of coordinating care. Clients often have multiple healthcare providers (primary care physician, orthopedist, endocrinologist, cardiologist) and may be prescribing different medications and treatments without adequate information about treatments prescribed by others, so the case manager must monitor all aspects of care and coordinate with all healthcare providers.

166. B: A concurrent review is generally carried out when a client is hospitalized in order to determine if the client is receiving an appropriate level of care. The case manager should interview the client and review the client's history and medical records. The concurrent review is utilized to determine whether or not a client needs to remain hospitalized or could be discharged or transferred to another level of care, such as to a subacute facility or skilled nursing facility.

167. C: If a client in an acute care hospital is stable but will require 7 further days of IV antibiotics during recovery from surgery and a severe post-operative infection, the most appropriate level of care is a subacute care facility. Subacute facilities are sometimes stand-alone facilities or a special unit in an acute care hospital. Subacute care is intended for clients who are stable but still have a need for ongoing in-patient care for a limited period of time.

168. D: If conducting a behavioral health assessment for a client who is noncompliant with treatment, the case manager should focus on the reason for the behavior rather the effects of how the behavior is exhibited. For example, the case manager should assess things as the cost of treatment and the ability of the client to pay, the time needed for compliance activities and the other responsibilities the client has (children, work) that may interfere, and access to transportation.

169. B: Insurance companies hire case managers primarily to reduce the costs of care. This does not mean that care is less than optimal but that the care that is provided is appropriate for the client's needs. This may mean that clients are transferred to a different level of care rather than staying in an acute hospital or are referred to a home health agency and discharged if care can be provided at lower cost in the home environment.

170. D: If a client's insurance is an exclusive provider organization (EPO) and the client chooses to see a physician outside of the network and receives a bill for $500, the client must pay 100%. With an EPO, there is no gatekeeper physician, so the client is able to make an appointment with a specialist without a referral, but the program limits coverage to those physicians who are contracted with the EPO except in the case of emergency. However, even with an emergency, once the client is stabilized, the client should be transferred to the care of physicians in the EPO; and this may require transfer to a different hospital.

171. C: The client who has been covered by an employer-sponsored insurance plan but is not qualified to apply for COBRA is a client who quit the job that covered the insurance. However, if the client had been laid off, divorced the primary insurance holder, or was the spouse of a primary insurance holder who died, the client is then qualified to apply for COBRA. Coverage can continue for from 18-36 months, but costs may be higher because the client has to cover the complete cost of the policy.

172. B: If a client on Medicare requires durable medical equipment, the costs should be covered by Medicare B, which also covers outpatient services, diagnostic tests, and home health care. Medicare A covers inpatient services, such as hospitalization, including different levels from acute to skilled nursing facilities and hospice and rehabilitation care. Medicare C covers services normally covered by Medicare A and B for Medicare Advantage plans. Medicare D is the prescription drug plan.

173. C: If a client is admitted to a skilled nursing facility (SNF) after a qualifying stay in an acute hospital, Medicare provides coverage for up to 100 days. However, the client must pay a copay after 20 days in the SNF. The client must be receiving medically-necessary care and must show progress during the stay at the SNF or the care is disallowed, and the client must be discharged or pay the entire cost of care. Medicare will not cover the cost of custodial care for clients whose primary need is assistance with ADLs.

174. B: In order for a client to qualify for Social Security Disability Insurance, the client or the person on whom the client is dependent must have been employed for at least 10 years. SSDI is intended for clients who are blind or otherwise permanently disabled and are unable to work because of the disability. The dollar amount of the SSDI payments is based on the salary received by the client or the person on whom the client is dependent. The client becomes eligible for Medicare, regardless of age, after 2 years on SSDI.

175. D: If a Medicare client does not meet the qualifications for SSDI but is 68 years old, low income, and disabled, the case manager should advise the client to apply for SSI (Supplemental Security Income), which provides cash benefits for clients who are 65 or older and blind or otherwise disabled but unlike SSDI has no employment requirement. Clients who qualify for SSI also automatically qualify for their states Medicaid program, which should cover the healthcare costs that Medicare does not cover. The client must apply for any other cash benefits to which the client may be eligible, such as pension plans and Social Security.

176. A: In order for a client to qualify for VA benefits, the client must have been honorably discharged and served on active duty for a minimum of 24 months. If a client received less than an honorable discharge, the person can apply for an upgrade, but the process for qualifying is lengthy and may require up to 12 months or more. If the client received less than an honorable discharge but is exhibiting health problems related to service (such as PTSD or other mental or physical health problem), the client is eligible for benefits immediately.

177. B: If a client was injured at work and is undergoing rehabilitation for physical strengthening 2 days a week in preparation for returning to work, this is referred to as work conditioning. Work hardening is more intensive and involves rehabilitation for 3 to 5 days a week. Work adjustment focuses on the skills and abilities the client will need to be successful at work. Some clients return to the job with transitional work duty; that is, the work load has been modified to fit the ability of the client.

178. A: To classify inpatients for reimbursement, Medicare utilizes MS-DRG (Medicare Severity Diagnosis-Related Groups). The MS-DRG is based on the client's primary and secondary diagnosis, surgical procedures scheduled during the hospitalization, and complications and comorbidities (CC) or major complications and comorbidities (MCC). Based on the client's assigned MS-DRG, the hospital receives a flat fee for client care. AP-DRG (All patient), IR-DRG (International refined), and APR-DRG (All Patient Refined) are diagnosis-related groups used by other organizations, such as insurance companies.

179. A: Storming. Tuckman's stages of group development:

- Forming: Leader takes active role and members follow.
- Storming: Opinions diverge and conflict may occur. Resistance may occur as shown by the absence of members, shared silence, and subgroup formation.
- Norming: Members begin to express positive feelings toward each other and feel attached to the group.
- Performing: Leader's input and direction decreases and focuses primarily on keeping the members on track with tasks.
- Mourning: The group disbands or leader/members leave the group.

180. C: The score for the REALM (Rapid Estimate of Adult Literacy in Medicine) test is based on the number of words the client can pronounce. The client is given a form with three different lists of medical terms in increasing difficulty from simple one syllable words (fat, flu, stress), to two (bowel, asthma, rectal), and to three and four (appendix, menopause, potassium, osteoporosis). The client reads the lists aloud and is allowed to skip unfamiliar words.

Practice Test #2

1. When choosing a community vendor to supply durable medical equipment (DME) to a client, the most important factor is:
- a. Reliability.
- b. Proximity.
- c. Quality.
- d. Cost.

2. When conducting a survey for program evaluation, the easiest questions to quantify are:
- a. Descriptive informational questions (who, what, when, where, how, how much, and why).
- b. Yes/no questions.
- c. Multiple-choice questions.
- d. Rating scale.

3. The primary purpose of the Caseload Matrix in caseload calculations is to:
- a. Differentiate activities and interventions.
- b. Measure specific outcomes.
- c. Determine accuracy of caseload calculations.
- d. Identify variables in various settings affecting caseloads.

4. Using the four-point Likert scale to assess clients with low self-care, a client with severe risk of failing to adhere to medical regimens/treatments is classified as:
- a. Level 1.
- b. Level 2.
- c. Level 3.
- d. Level 4.

5. A young adult in the emergency department for attempted suicide with three previous attempts should be:
- a. Referred to outpatient mental health services.
- b. Treated and discharged to family.
- c. Asked to sign a "no-suicide contract" before discharge.
- d. Admitted to the hospital.

6. The three-midnight rule for extended Medicare benefit applies to clients transferring to:
- a. Skilled nursing facilities.
- b. Home health agency services.
- c. Long-term care facilities for rehabilitation.
- d. Assisted living facilities.

7. The InterQual utilization management tool, which is used to determine if interventions are appropriate and properly sequenced, is considered to be:
- a. A retrospective monitoring tool.
- b. Clinical evidence summaries.
- c. Level-of-care criteria tools.
- d. Care-planning criteria tools.

8. Identifying the need for environmental modifications in a client's home is a role of the certified case manager (CCM) under the domain of:

    a. Outcomes evaluation/case closure.
    b. Utilization management.
    c. Vocational concepts and strategies.
    d. Clinical care management.

9. A set of expected behaviors and consequences related to a case manager's place in a particular social structure, such as an acute hospital, is a:

    a. Process.
    b. Role.
    c. Activity.
    d. Function.

10. Under the CMS Quality Framework for Home and Community Based Services, participant safeguards include:

    a. Licensure and certification of staff.
    b. Right to make decisions.
    c. Incident reporting.
    d. Surveys of outcomes.

11. The most significant challenge to community-based case managers is:

    a. The acutely ill.
    b. Pediatric clients.
    c. Mothers and infants.
    d. The chronically ill.

12. The primary purpose of negotiation in case management practice is to:

    a. Control costs and provide medically necessary services.
    b. Avoid conflict and promote cooperation.
    c. Educate participants.
    d. Represent the payor's interests.

13. A requirement for participation in a pharmacy assistance program usually includes:

    a. Prescription insurance coverage or Medicare D.
    b. Generic prescriptions only.
    c. U.S. residency.
    d. Income of less than 200% of federal poverty level.

14. Under InterQual's ISD criteria of severity of illness (SI) reflecting the need for acute hospitalization, onset of symptoms within one week is categorized as:

    a. Acute/sudden onset.
    b. Recently or newly discovered.
    c. Recent onset.
    d. Newly discovered.

15. With mandatory beneficiary ownership of capped rental durable medical equipment (DME), once ownership has passed to the beneficiary, Medicare will pay for:

 a. Routine service and maintenance.
 b. Only repairs necessary to make the DME serviceable.
 c. All routine service and repairs.
 d. No service or repairs.

16. The best placement for a 47-year-old male with an IQ of 68 who cannot live alone is probably a:

 a. Group home.
 b. Skilled nursing facility.
 c. Assisted living facility.
 d. Mental health facility.

17. Denial or noncertification of services may result from:

 a. Extended hospitalization because of postoperative myocardial infarction.
 b. Extended hospitalization because PT is not available on weekends.
 c. Change in policy after services rendered.
 d. Client's death.

18. If a client in an acute hospital has comorbidities of prostate cancer, Type 1 diabetes, hypertension, and pneumonia, the priority in treatment is:

 a. Prostate cancer.
 b. Type 1 diabetes.
 c. Hypertension.
 d. Pneumonia.

19. The average length of stay (LOS) in an acute hospital for a complete knee replacement is approximately:

 a. 3 days.
 b. 4 days.
 c. 7 days.
 d. 10 days.

20. If a client has outpatient surgery in the morning and stays overnight for extended observation, the client becomes an inpatient:

 a. At midnight.
 b. After 8 hours.
 c. When the physician orders inpatient services.
 d. After 24 hours.

21. A case manager in the emergency department (ED) must consider national indicators for ED crowding, such as:

 a. Need for follow-up appointments.
 b. Acute hospital admission.
 c. Diversions.
 d. Unsafe discharges.

22. The case manager in the admitting department serves essentially as a:

   a. Gatekeeper.
   b. Negotiator.
   c. Communicator.
   d. Supervisor.

23. When a client is receiving occupational therapy in the home, documentation must include:

   a. Costs.
   b. Client preferences.
   c. Realistic and measurable goals.
   d. Indirect supervision of unlicensed staff.

24. The best initial method of ensuring correct medication dosage for a home client who wants to remain independent but sometimes forgets to take her morning medications or takes a double dose is:

   a. Hiring an aide to come in daily to give medications.
   b. Providing an electronic alarmed medication delivery device.
   c. Placing the client in an assisted living facility.
   d. Arranging for someone to telephone daily.

25. The Older Americans Act provides:

   a. Hospital services.
   b. Pharmacy assistance programs.
   c. Home and community services.
   d. Financial assistance to older adults.

26. Initial symptom management of shortness of breath in a palliative care client usually includes:

   a. Elevating the head and using a fan aimed toward the person's face.
   b. Corticosteroids.
   c. Oxygen by nasal cannula.
   d. Bronchodilators.

27. In Kurt Lewin's change theory, the first stage, motivation to change, is also referred to as:

   a. Freezing.
   b. Unfreezing.
   c. Unfrozen.
   d. Refreezing.

28. A person who is resistive to seeing a psychologist for severe emotional problems because of a personal belief that prayer will heal may benefit most from:

   a. Pastoral counseling.
   b. Personal meditation.
   c. Medications.
   d. Spiritual instructions.

29. For a trauma patient who will need long-term care and has no coverage and no financial resources beyond Social Security income, the acute care case manager should explore:

    a. Charity organizations.
    b. Extended acute care.
    c. Home health agency care.
    d. State long-term care programs.

30. To facilitate the continuum of care after a client is discharged from an acute hospital, the most important relationship for a case manager to develop is with:

    a. Physician's staff.
    b. HMO clinicians.
    c. Skilled nursing facilities and home health agencies.
    d. Acute hospital administrators.

31. A tool that provides a client's self-assessment of functional health and quality-of-life issues is the:

    a. Health Status Survey (SF-36).
    b. Patient Health Questionnaire (PHQ).
    c. Post Deployment Clinical Assessment Tool (PDCAT).
    d. Barthel Index.

32. The type of group therapy that aims to help members who share a common problem learn to cope is:

    a. Education group.
    b. Self-help group.
    c. Psychotherapy group.
    d. Support group.

33. The national organization that may provide the best information for the family of a young man who suffered a third concussion as a football injury is:

    a. American College of Sports Medicine.
    b. American Association of Physical Medicine and Rehabilitation.
    c. Brain Trauma Foundation.
    d. Orthopedic Research Society.

34. The primary purpose of a health coach is to:

    a. Prescribe treatment.
    b. Guide clients to discuss concerns regarding recovery.
    c. Counsel clients.
    d. Ensure treatment compliance.

35. The best intervention for a 68-year-old male with COPD who lives alone and manages his own care but has been eating only candy and snack foods is:

    a. Nutritional counseling.
    b. Admission to assisted-living facility.
    c. Home delivery of meals (Meals On Wheels).
    d. Referral to an occupational therapist.

36. The first step in crisis intervention is:
  a. Devising a plan.
  b. Assessing the problem and the triggering event.
  c. Teaching coping mechanisms.
  d. Evaluating resources.

37. Older adults with chronic illnesses that result in pain and/or physical limitations should often be evaluated for:
  a. Dementia.
  b. Depression.
  c. Drug abuse.
  d. Alcoholism.

38. The coping mechanism that involves actively searching for a way to reduce stress and cope is:
  a. Problem solving.
  b. Avoidance.
  c. Physical activity.
  d. Spirituality.

39. The best response to a dying Hmong patient who states that a shaman is coming to heal her is:
  a. "That is not realistic in your condition."
  b. "If you believe, then a cure is possible."
  c. "You will need your doctor's permission."
  d. "What can I do to help?"

40. For a person with a dual diagnosis, the initial treatment usually focuses on:
  a. Detoxification.
  b. Rehabilitation.
  c. Mental health treatment.
  d. Coping strategies.

41. Health literacy primarily requires:
  a. Basic reading, numerical, and comprehension, and communications skills.
  b. A thorough understanding of disease and appropriate treatments.
  c. An above-average intellectual capacity.
  d. Motivation to learn about health.

42. Bereavement is:
  a. A normal response to loss.
  b. The public expression of grief.
  c. Change of mood and feeling of sadness.
  d. The time period of mourning.

43. An alert elderly home care patient who complains that items have begun disappearing from her home is most likely the victim of:

    a. Elder abuse.
    b. Psychological abuse.
    c. Financial abuse.
    d. Physical abuse.

44. Before making a telephone call to a client to review status, the case manager should:

    a. Prepare a script.
    b. Outline the objectives of the call.
    c. Send a mail notification.
    d. Notify the physician.

45. Under the Case Management Society of America (CMSA) Standards of Practice, the standard of Facilitation, Coordination, and Collaboration can be demonstrated by:

    a. Documentation of termination of care.
    b. Documentation of ongoing efforts at collaboration with the client.
    c. Use of screening for high-risk individuals.
    d. Use of mediation/negotiation.

46. If all shelters are full and an indigent uninsured client with planned discharge in three days is placed on a waiting list for a preferred shelter, then the case manager's next action should be to:

    a. Call daily to determine where the client is on the list.
    b. Place the client on a second waiting list.
    c. Plan transfer to a skilled nursing facility until shelter placement is possible.
    d. Refer the problem to social services.

47. Bloodshot eyes, sniffing repeatedly, altered sleeping habits, and marked weight loss are indications of:

    a. Excess smoking.
    b. Cocaine abuse.
    c. Alcoholism.
    d. Marijuana abuse.

48. For a patient recovering from a brain injury, the Glasgow coma score that indicates potential for rehabilitation is:

    a. 3.
    b. 5.
    c. 8.
    d. 10.

49. Upon discharge from an acute hospital, the most appropriate placement for a client who has slight dementia and requires a simple daily dry dressing change but is medically stable and ambulates independently with a cane is:

    a. Subacute/rehabilitation facility.
    b. Skilled nursing facility.
    c. Intermediate care facility.
    d. Assisted living/custodial care facility.

50. An example of unskilled care is:

    a. Administering sliding scale insulin.
    b. Instructing a client on a low-sodium diet.
    c. Instructions in the use of assistive devices.
    d. Taking and reporting routine vital signs.

51. A client's or parent's refusal of care may be overridden if:

    a. The physician orders the care provided despite client objections.
    b. The client is mentally incompetent.
    c. The patient is elderly.
    d. The client is a minor child.

52. A risk factor for malnutrition is:

    a. Poverty.
    b. Recent weight loss of five pounds.
    c. Recent weight gain of five to eight pounds.
    d. Dentures.

53. A psychosocial evaluation is indicated for a client with:

    a. Chronic heart disease.
    b. Homelessness.
    c. Unintentional overdose.
    d. Limited financial resources.

54. The legal element of negligence that refers to a failure to carry out duties in accordance with accepted and usual standards of practice is:

    a. Duty.
    b. Breach.
    c. Causation.
    d. Harm.

55. Job accommodations for an office worker with fine motor impairment might include:

    a. Providing speech recognition program for computer access.
    b. Modifying the workstation to increase accessibility.
    c. Providing stand/lean stools.
    d. Providing rolling safety ladders.

56. During case selection, the client that is most likely to need and benefit from case management services is:

    a. 12-year-old child having a tonsillectomy.
    b. 67-year-old man having a transurethral resection of the prostate (TURP).
    c. 47-year-old Type 2 diabetic with severe insulin reaction after a bout of food poisoning with vomiting and diarrhea.
    d. 72-year-old woman with a postoperative wound infection after hip replacement.

57. When a facility is converting to the interoperable electronic healthcare delivery system, the most important aspect to consider is:

    a. Equipment choice.
    b. Time needed for conversion.
    c. Staff training.
    d. Staff preference.

58. The client-centered model of care in which a primary care physician manages, facilitates, and coordinates all levels of client care, including care provided by specialists, is:

    a. Chronic care model.
    b. Medical home model.
    c. Planned care model.
    d. Expanded care model.

59. Using real tasks or simulated work-related tasks and progressive exercises to strengthen and condition a person to return to work is an example of:

    a. Job coaching.
    b. Work adjustment.
    c. Transitional employment.
    d. Work hardening.

60. A client being discharged from an acute hospital with an infusion pump for multiple intravenous medications can be transferred to:

    a. Subacute and rehabilitation facilities.
    b. Skilled nursing facility.
    c. Subacute and skilled nursing facilities.
    d. Intermediate care facility.

61. During assessment and problem identification for a client with multiple physicians, if inconsistencies in medical data are found, the case manager should first:

    a. Consult with the client.
    b. Accept the latest information as most accurate.
    c. Consult with the source of inconsistent data.
    d. Ask for a medical review of client care.

62. The level of care that provides people with moderate assistance in activities of daily living and periodic nursing supervision for some activities is:

    a. Custodial care.
    b. Intermediate care.
    c. Skilled nursing.
    d. Acute care.

63. Criteria for Medicare coverage of home oxygen for a client receiving oxygen at 5L/min includes drawing arterial blood gases while the client:

    a. Receives oxygen at 5L/min.
    b. Receives oxygen at <3L/min.
    c. Receives oxygen at 4L/min.
    d. Breathes room air.

64. The correct elbow angle for an officer worker when sitting in a chair and using a computer keyboard is:

    a. 45 degrees.
    b. 60 degrees.
    c. 90 degrees.
    d. 120 degrees.

65. Durable medical equipment (DME) such as shower chairs and handrails are further classified as:

    a. Mobility aids.
    b. Assistive devices.
    c. High-tech equipment.
    d. Cognitive aids.

66. Underutilization may result from:

    a. Delays in performing necessary diagnostic procedures.
    b. Client's insistence on expensive procedures.
    c. Client's being in a teaching hospital.
    d. Physician's concern about liability.

67. The type of insurance plan that offers the most flexibility is the:

    a. Health maintenance organizations.
    b. Managed indemnity plans.
    c. Indemnity plans.
    d. Point-of-service plans.

68. Under utilization management services, the review that determines whether hospitalization is justified is:

    a. Telephonic review.
    b. Retrospective review.
    c. Concurrent review.
    d. Prospective review.

69. When conflicts arise over coverage for treatment, the case manager's primary responsibility is to:

    a. The payor.
    b. The client.
    c. The utilization review committee.
    d. The care provider.

70. The National Quality Forum (NQF) measures that determine if correct actions, such as cervical cancer screening, have been completed are:

    a. Process measures.
    b. Outcomes measures.
    c. Patient experience measures.
    d. Structural measures.

71. The Instrumental Activities of Daily Living (IADL) tool includes assessment of:

    a. Bathing.

    b. Toileting.

    c. Ascending or descending stairs.

    d. Financial responsibility.

72. The type of variance that occurs when durable medical equipment for home care is unavailable is:

    a. Community variance.

    b. Practitioner variance.

    c. Institution/systems variance.

    d. Client/family variance.

73. The type of assessment that evaluates hazards in the home, such as loose carpets, rotting food, or piles of paper on the floor, is:

    a. Physical assessment.

    b. Functional assessment.

    c. Environmental assessment.

    d. Psychosocial assessment.

74. A learner outcome for teaching diabetics about insulin reaction is:

    a. Identify different types of insulin.

    b. List and describe the symptoms of insulin reaction.

    c. Identify foods high in carbohydrates.

    d. Explain the difference between Type 1 and Type 2 diabetes.

75. Case management differs from managed care in that case management is primarily:

    a. People-oriented.

    b. Systems-oriented.

    c. Regulation-oriented.

    d. Nursing-oriented.

76. After complicated labor and Caesarean, a woman must be covered for hospitalization by her insurance carrier for:

    a. 24 hours.

    b. 96 hours.

    c. 48 hours.

    d. 36 hours.

77. For employment experience to be accepted for CM certification, the applicant must:

    a. Perform at least six or eight essential activities related to client contact.

    b. Be licensed or certified to practice independently.

    c. Practice case management at least 25% of the time.

    d. Perform work in at least four of six core components of case management.

78. A Medicare client who was hospitalized for a brain injury may be eligible for home health care to provide:

a. Nursing care 24 hours a day.
b. Home-delivered meals.
c. Personal care (bathing, dressing) alone.
d. Occupational therapy.

79. When evaluating outcomes data for evidence-based practice, the type of data that includes measures of mortality, longevity, and cost-effectiveness is:

a. Clinical.
b. Psychosocial.
c. Integrative.
d. Physiological.

80. The primary focus of Workers' Compensation is to:

a. Prevent economic hardship.
b. Return people to work.
c. Contain costs.
d. Promote workers' safety.

81. A case mix group, as defined by the Health Insurance Prospective Payment System (HIPPS), is:

a. A classification system based on utilization of resources.
b. A data set containing elements to review for a comprehensive assessment of client function.
c. A classification system based on clinical characteristics of clients.
d. A data set used by home health agencies to measure outcomes and risk factors.

82. If a client has insurance from a self-funded, employer-sponsored health plan and questions of coverage arise, the case manager should contact:

a. The plan's benefit manager.
b. The employer.
c. The client.
d. The physician.

83. The primary purpose of pharmacy benefit management is to:

a. Increase use of generic drugs.
b. Reduce costs of drugs.
c. Promote drug safety.
d. Provide a drug formulary for clients.

84. The level of independence or care in the home for an adult female indicated by a discharge Functional Independence Measure (FIM™) score of 63, with scores in all areas ranging from 3 to 4 is:

a. Complete independence in care.
b. Modified independence, including use of assistive devices and activity modification.
c. Supervision only (standby without physically assisting).
d. Minimal to moderate contact assistance (physically assisting).

85. The first step in doing a cultural assessment is:
   a. Explain the purpose of a cultural assessment.
   b. Ask permission to do a cultural assessment.
   c. Take thorough notes during communication.
   d. Establish trust.

86. Intensive case management for assertive community treatment is focused on providing care for:
   a. Brain injuries.
   b. Mental health issues.
   c. Spinal cord injuries.
   d. Alzheimer's disease.

87. Palliative care can begin when:
   a. A client is diagnosed with a life-threatening disease.
   b. A client's life expectancy is less than one year.
   c. A client's life expectancy is six months or less.
   d. A client requests palliative care.

88. When healthcare providers disagree about the best plan of care, the first step in resolving this conflict is to:
   a. Allow both individuals to present their side of the conflict without bias.
   b. Encourage them to reach a compromise.
   c. Tell them they are violating professional standards of conduct.
   d. Make a decision about the matter.

89. According to the Consolidated Omnibus Budget Reconciliation Act (COBRA), the usual duration for which an ex-employee may have continued insurance coverage is:
   a. 12 months.
   b. 18 months.
   c. 24 months.
   d. 36 months.

90. The primary criterion for referral to a hospice program is:
   a. Severe intractable pain.
   b. Life-threatening disease.
   c. Probability that death will occur within six months.
   d. DNR order.

91. An example of hard savings that can result from case management is:
   a. Avoiding hospital readmission.
   b. Avoiding home health care.
   c. Preventing medical errors.
   d. Changing length of stay.

92. The most appropriate addition to an interdisciplinary care team (ICT) to assist in coordinating care for increasing numbers of pediatric clients would be:

    a. Child life specialist.
    b. Occupational therapist.
    c. Dietitian.
    d. Play therapist.

93. When determining the burden of proof for acts of negligence, risk management would classify willfully providing inadequate care while disregarding the safety and security of another as:

    a. Negligent conduct.
    b. Gross negligence.
    c. Contributory negligence.
    d. Comparative negligence.

94. If the case manager at a hospital determines that a client does not need a discharge plan for transition of care, but the physician orders one, the hospital:

    a. Can choose to omit the discharge plan.
    b. Must develop the plan.
    c. May develop a simplified discharge plan.
    d. May substitute with general information materials.

95. A legal document that specifically designates someone to make decisions regarding medical and end-of-life care if a client is mentally incompetent is a(n):

    a. Advance directive.
    b. Do-not-resuscitate order.
    c. Durable power of attorney.
    d. General power of attorney.

96. If two clients need a hospital bed, but only one is available, the decision regarding which client to transfer should be based on the ethical principle of:

    a. Nonmaleficence.
    b. Beneficence.
    c. Justice.
    d. Autonomy.

97. The theory that states that a change in one family member's behavior will affect others in the family is:

    a. Health Belief Model (Rosenstock).
    b. Theory of Planned Behavior (Ajzen).
    c. Family Systems Theory (Bowen).
    d. Theory of Reasoned Action (Fishbein and Ajzen).

98. Kolb's model of experiential learning is best described as:

    a. Knowledge develops from experience interacting with cognition and perception.
    b. Knowledge and experience are equally important.
    c. Experience precedes knowledge in learning.
    d. Learning cannot be acquired without experience and perception.

99. When a client's spouse asks for information about another client, the response that complies with the Health Insurance Portability and Accountability Act (HIPAA) is:

    a. "The law doesn't allow me to give out any information about clients in order to protect their privacy and safety."
    b. "His wife is in the lounge. You can go ask her."
    c. "Why are you asking?"
    d. "He has bipolar disease, like your husband."

100. A prevention strategy that encourages physicians, nurses, and other healthcare providers to discuss smoking cessation with all adolescents is an example of:

    a. Secondary prevention.
    b. Universal primary prevention.
    c. Indicated primary prevention.
    d. Targeted primary prevention.

101. The method used to determine monetary savings resulting from planned interventions is:

    a. Cost/benefit analysis.
    b. Cost-effective analysis.
    c. Efficacy study.
    d. Cost/utility analysis.

102. For quality/performance improvement, the best tool to determine methods to streamline processes is:

    a. Root cause analysis.
    b. Tracer methodology.
    c. Family survey.
    d. Staff survey.

103. A violation of professional boundaries on the part of the case manager is:

    a. Accepting a box of chocolates to be shared by all unit staff from a client's daughter.
    b. Confiding to the client that he, like the client, is getting a divorce, so he understands the client's stress.
    c. Assisting a client in placing a call to his landlord so the client can explain that he cannot pay the rent on time.
    d. Noticing that a client is crying and placing his hand on the client's shoulder.

104. The most critical skill for a case manager collaborating in an interdisciplinary team is:

    a. Patience.
    b. Assertiveness.
    c. Empathy with others.
    d. Willingness to compromise.

105. If a 24-year-old Asian client states a treatment preference but plans to leave the decision to her family members, the case manager should:

    a. Try to convince the client to assert herself.
    b. Recognize that cultural values regarding individualism vary, and respect the client's right to be guided by family.
    c. Tell the family that the client should be the one to make the decision.
    d. Ask the ethics committee to intervene.

106. The following act prevents transfer of a client from the ED until the client stabilizes:

    a. The Health Insurance Portability and Accountability Act (HIPAA).
    b. The Emergency Medical Treatment and Active Labor Act (EMTALA).
    c. Americans with Disabilities Act (ADA).
    d. Older Americans Act (OAA).

107. An example of documentation that is currently on The Joint Commission's "Do Not Use" list is:

    a. 5 mg.
    b. 0.5 mg.
    c. 15 U.
    d. @.

108. If all clients who develop urinary infections with urinary catheters are evaluated per urine culture and sensitivities for microbial resistance, but only those clients with clinically evident infections are included, this is an example of:

    a. Information bias.
    b. Selection bias.
    c. Compliance bias.
    d. Admission bias.

109. The National Patient Safety Goals communication requirements related to telephone orders or reporting include:

    a. The receiver "reading back" the orders or report.
    b. The receiver repeating each part of an order or report as it's given.
    c. The individual giving orders or reports asks if information understood.
    d. The individual giving orders or reports repeats each item twice.

110. A necessary component of informed consent prior to a procedure is:

    a. Names of assisting staff members.
    b. Beginning and ending times.
    c. Risks and benefits of the procedure.
    d. Facility statistics regarding the procedure.

111. When instituting a plan for risk management, the primary concern in the statement of purpose should be:

    a. Reduction in financial risk.
    b. Client safety.
    c. Decreased liability.
    d. Scope of program.

112. The Mini-Cog Test to assess for dementia includes:

    a. Counting backward from 100 by 7s.
    b. Copying a picture of interlocking shapes.
    c. Following simple three-part directions.
    d. Drawing the face of a clock with the hands indicating a specified time.

113. Outcomes are derived from:

    a. Client, nurse, and system.
    b. Client only.
    c. Clients, physicians, and nurses.
    d. Nurse only.

114. A community resource that can provide nursing and personal care in the home is:

    a. Public health department.
    b. Home health agency.
    c. Social services.
    d. Senior citizens' organization.

115. The primary focus of a risk mitigation program is:

    a. To decrease adverse patient outcomes and reduce liability.
    b. To improve processes of care.
    c. To improve patient outcomes.
    d. To adhere to professional standards.

116. The governmental agency responsible for bloodborne pathogens standards in medical institutions is:

    a. CDC.
    b. OSHA.
    c. EPA.
    d. FDA.

117. With the continuous quality improvement (CQI) model, the focus of improvement is on:

    a. Processes.
    b. Staff.
    c. Administrative personnel.
    d. Clients.

118. When developing guidelines for evidence-based practice, the weakest justification for establishing a procedure is:

    a. Evidence review.
    b. Staff preference.
    c. Policy considerations.
    d. Expert judgment.

119. Viatical settlements primarily benefit:

    a. Beneficiaries.
    b. Healthcare providers.
    c. Insurance companies.
    d. Policyholders.

120. The model for managed care that provides services at discounted rates to those enrolled is:

a. Health maintenance organization (HMO).
b. Point of service plan (POS).
c. Preferred provider organization (PPO).
d. Exclusive provider organization (EPO).

121. The model for health maintenance organizations in which the HMO hires physicians to work in clinic-type settings is:

a. Group model.
b. Network model.
c. Staff model.
d. Direct contact model.

122. Medicare B benefits include:

a. Hospitalization (acute care).
b. Skilled nursing facility care.
c. Clinical laboratory services.
d. Hospice care.

123. The healthcare insurance reimbursement system that involves an advanced fixed monthly payment to a provider is:

a. Per-diem reimbursement.
b. Fee-for-service.
c. Pay-for-performance.
d. Capitation.

124. The Agency for Healthcare Research and Quality (AHRQ)'s Quality Indicators (QIs) that measure the quality of care for disorders sensitive to outpatient care (with good care reducing the need for hospitalization) are:

a. Prevention QIs.
b. Inpatient QIs.
c. Patient safety indicators (PSIs).
d. Pediatric QIs.

125. Core measures for Centers for Medicare & Medicaid Services (CMS) include measures related to:

a. Cancer.
b. Brain injuries.
c. Asthma care for children.
d. Alzheimer's disease.

126. URAC case management accreditation standards require healthcare organizations, such as managed care programs, to establish processes to:

a. Assess, plan, and implement case management interventions.
b. Evaluate outcomes of case management interventions.
c. Conduct peer reviews of case management interventions.
d. Cut costs of case management interventions.

127. The healthcare accreditation agency that assists purchasers of health plans and consumers to evaluate the performance of health plans is:
    a. Centers for Medicare & Medicaid Services (CMS).
    b. The Joint Commission (formerly JCAHO).
    c. URAC.
    d. National Committee for Quality Assurance (NCQA).

128. The government agency that regulates protection of human subjects involved in research projects for experimental treatments is:
    a. FDA.
    b. OSHA.
    c. CMS.
    d. CDC.

129. Eligibility criteria for Supplemental Security Income (SSI) for those with low income and few resources include:
    a. Deafness.
    b. Age 55 or older.
    c. Chronic pain.
    d. Blindness.

130. Guidelines for eligibility and reimbursement in Medicaid programs are established by:
    a. The Social Security Administration.
    b. Individual counties.
    c. State consortia.
    d. Individual states.

131. Under the chronic care model, the primary purpose of utilizing community resources is to:
    a. Identify client needs.
    b. Improve client's self-management skills.
    c. Reduce the need for rehospitalization.
    d. Reduce costs.

132. If a client has only Medicare and no supplementary insurance and her physician accepts Medicare, the client's out-of-pocket cost for care will be:
    a. Nothing.
    b. 10%.
    c. 20%.
    d. 80%.

133. A client with both Tricare and Medicare may avoid hospitalization in a Veterans' Affairs medical facility because:
    a. Tricare and Medicare combined reimburse for only 80% of costs.
    b. The VA can bill neither Tricare nor Medicare.
    c. The VA cannot bill Tricare.
    d. The VA cannot bill Medicare.

134. Criteria for Social Security Disability Insurance (SSDI) include a physical/mental disability as well as:
   a. Restriction in employment ability.
   b. Age >65.
   c. Limited income.
   d. Expectation of permanent disability.

135. A specified dollar amount that a client must pay at the time of receiving healthcare services is a:
   a. Premium.
   b. Copayment.
   c. Deductible.
   d. Coinsurance.

136. If a child has been hospitalized three times in 12 months with acute asthma because of noncompliance with the treatment regimen, the best initial action of the case manager is:
   a. Make a referral to child protective services (CPS).
   b. Reprimand the parents.
   c. Suggest a change in treatment regimen.
   d. Question the reasons for noncompliance.

137. An affidavit of merit is usually filed to:
   a. Support a lawsuit for malpractice.
   b. Refute a lawsuit for malpractice.
   c. Reward excellence in service.
   d. Confer accreditation.

138. The most appropriate rehabilitation placement for a 72-year-old woman who lives alone and had a hip replacement five days earlier is:
   a. Rehabilitation in an acute hospital.
   b. Rehabilitation in the provider's office.
   c. Rehabilitation in her home.
   d. Rehabilitation in a skilled nursing/rehabilitation facility.

139. For a client with peripheral arterial disease (PAD), an ankle-brachial index (ABI) score of 0.37 indicates
   a. A limb-threatening condition, with pain at rest.
   b. Mild narrowing of one or more blood vessels.
   c. A normal reading, likely asymptomatic.
   d. Possible calcification of vessel walls.

140. For a client with a chronic mental health disorder, recovery means:
   a. Absence of symptoms.
   b. Discontinuation of mental health service.
   c. Coping with symptoms and problems.
   d. Independence in meeting individual needs.

141. Client empowerment primarily requires:

    a. Options, authority, and action.
    b. Time and effort.
    c. Intellectual capacity.
    d. Institutional support.

142. Threatening to injure and withhold food and clothes from a person who is uncooperative is an example of:

    a. Physical abuse.
    b. Psychological abuse.
    c. Neglect.
    d. Financial abuse.

143. Medication reconciliation should be completed:

    a. Prior to admission.
    b. During the admission assessment.
    c. On discharge.
    d. During all phases of care.

144. If the case manager observes an elderly patient in an assisted living facility is unkempt, dehydrated, and fearful and has a number of unexplained bruises, the case manager's most appropriate response is to:

    a. Notify the owner of the facility.
    b. Reprimand caregivers.
    c. Notify appropriate state authorities, such as adult protective services.
    d. Arrange for transfer to another facility.

145. According to InterQual's ISD discharge reviews, the appropriate discharge documentation of a client admitted with a WBC of 15,000 and temperature of 39.8 °C is:

    a. "Client stable."
    b. "Infection cleared."
    c. "Client's laboratory findings and temperature within normal limits."
    d. "WBC 7,000 and temperature 37 °C."

146. An important purpose of a critical pathway is to:

    a. Allow flexibility.
    b. Focus on one discipline.
    c. Establish accountability.
    d. Reduce/prevent variations in care.

147. The first step in negotiation for a case manager should be:

    a. Statement of problem.
    b. Discussion.
    c. Research.
    d. Statement of financial limits.

148. A case manager who is contracted by an individual or family to manage healthcare needs and services is a(n):

    a. Private case manager.
    b. Independent case manager.
    c. Community-based case manager.
    d. Internal case manager.

149. The Milliman care guidelines that can be used for clients with very complex medical situations that do not easily fit into other guidelines are:

    a. General recovery guidelines.
    b. Inpatient and surgical care guidelines.
    c. Chronic care guidelines.
    d. Ambulatory care guidelines.

150. According to Tuckman's group developmental stages, the stage in which members express positive feelings toward each other is:

    a. Forming.
    b. Storming.
    c. Norming.
    d. Performing.

151. If a client recently discharged from rehabilitation for substance abuse calls the case manager crying and states she is going to kill herself, the best response is to:

    a. Advise the client to hang up and call the suicide prevention line.
    b. Conclude the call and call 9-1-1.
    c. Keep the client on the line and ask another individual to call 9-1-1.
    d. Put the client on hold and call 9-1-1.

152. If a mental health client must attend court-ordered Alcoholics Anonymous® (AA) meetings but tells the case manager that it's a waste of his time and that he is only going because he is forced to because he doesn't have a drinking problem, the most appropriate response is:

    a. "You should try to benefit from the meetings."
    b. "It's good that you are attending regularly."
    c. "AA can help you accept that you have a drinking problem."
    d. "You were driving drunk, so you do have a problem."

153. If the case manager is evaluating the facility's assessments and polices for fall risks in response to a suit against the facility for a client injury, the type of indicator the case manager is researching is a:

    a. Clinical indicator.
    b. Financial indicator.
    c. Productivity indicator.
    d. Quality indicator.

154. A factor that is not generally part of caseload calculation is:
a. Client acuity.
b. Practice setting.
c. Risk stratification.
d. Client gender.

155. When considering the cost effectiveness of case management, soft savings can include:
a. A client who transferred from an acute care hospital to a skilled nursing facility.
b. A client who loses weight and controls diabetes, resulting in fewer emergency room visits.
c. A client who switches from brand name medications to generic.
d. A client who stops curative treatments and enters hospice care.

156. If a client is transferred from an acute care hospital to an inpatient rehabilitation center, the client must be able to participate in therapy for a minimum of:
a. 1 hour daily.
b. 3 hours daily.
c. 5 hours daily.
d. 6 hours daily.

157. If a 56-year-old client has recovered well from a heart attack and is to undergo cardiac rehabilitation, the best option for the client is likely:
a. Outpatient rehabilitation program.
b. Inpatient rehabilitation center.
c. Subacute care facility.
d. Skilled nursing facility.

158. If a 46-year-old client with cerebral palsy receiving SSDI and Medicare has not worked for pay for 8 years but is interested in doing computer work from home using assistive devices, the case manager should advise the client that:
a. He would lose all of his government benefits if he is employed.
b. He should apply to the Ticket to Work program.
c. Reapplying is a difficult process if he can no longer work.
d. There are few jobs that involve working from home.

159. Under the Affordable Care Act, a benefit that is not part of the 10 essential benefits that must be covered each year by insurance companies without a dollar cap is:
a. Prescription drugs.
b. Laboratory services.
c. Dental care (Adult).
d. Maternity and Newborn care.

160. If a laptop computer with FIPS140-2 encryption was stolen from the case manager's car and contained PHI regarding clients, the case manager should:
a. Gather documents proving encryption.
b. Notify HHS of a breach of unsecured PHI.
c. Notify clients of a violation of privacy.
d. Place a media notice regarding the breach.

161. The situation that is not covered by the Family and Medical Leave Act is:

    a. The client's spouse wants family leave to care for the client during a short-term illness.
    b. The client wants medical leave because of a high-risk pregnancy.
    c. The client wants medical leave because of cancer treatment.
    d. A sibling wants family leave to care for the client during a serious illness.

162. If the client chooses to forego transfer to an inpatient rehabilitation center and have home health care instead against the advice of the physician and the case manager, and the case manager alters the plan of care to correspond with the client's wishes, the case manager is exhibiting the ethical principle of:

    a. Beneficence.
    b. Autonomy.
    c. Nonmaleficence.
    d. Justice.

163. If a deaf client who prefers to use sign language but can read and type is in a rehabilitation center away from family and friends, the best way for them to communicate is via:

    a. Teletypewriter (TTY).
    b. Messaging.
    c. Video chat (Facetime, Skype).
    d. E-mail.

164. A verbal exchange with a client should be documented as:

    a. "Client angry and uncooperative."
    b. "Client states treatment is not working and, therefore, refused to take medications."
    c. "Client refusing treatment, including medications."
    d. "Client appears upset with the medical care received."

165. When considering whether the Americans with Disabilities Act will provide protections for a client, the case manager recognizes that a condition that is not considered a disability is:

    a. Muscular dystrophy.
    b. HIV/AIDS.
    c. Transsexualism.
    d. Blindness.

166. The case manager uses Interqual®, an evidence-based tool, in order to determine:

    a. The client's level of acuity and level of care needed.
    b. The client's long-term risk factors.
    c. The estimated costs of client care.
    d. The client's eligibility for assistance programs.

167. The assessment that must be included in the Inpatient Rehabilitation Facility Patient Assessment Instrument (IRF-PAI) for CMS to determine the rate of payment for fee-for-service clients is:

    a. Mini-Mental State Exam (MMSE).
    b. Instrumental Activities of Daily Living (IADL).
    c. Index of Independence of Activities of Daily Living (Katz Index).
    d. Functional Independence Measure™ (FIM™).

168. If the case manager is utilizing the strengths model of case management, the case manager must assist the client to:

    a. Take responsibility for his/her own recovery.
    b. Identify family and friends who can serve as resources for recovery.
    c. Learn to manage self-care independently and decrease dependence on others.
    d. Identify abilities, skills, and environmental factors that may promote recovery.

169. If the case manager wants to make a change in procedures but concedes to another team member who opposes the changes, the approach to negotiation that the case manager is using is:

    a. Competition.
    b. Avoidance.
    c. Accommodation.
    d. Compromise.

170. If an Inpatient Prospective Patient System hospital in the Hospital Readmissions Reduction Program, the hospital is penalized if a client has an unplanned readmission for a condition included in the program within:

    a. 10 days.
    b. 15 days.
    c. 20 days.
    d. 30 days.

171. If a client with repeated emergency department visits for migraine headaches has received relief from a new treatment, but the client's insurance does not yet cover the cost of the very expensive medication and denied an appeal, the case manager should advise the client to:

    a. Pay privately for the medication.
    b. Apply to the pharmaceutical company's patient assistance program.
    c. Set up a Go-Fund-Me page for assistance.
    d. Try other medications and treatments.

172. If the case manager is utilizing video calls with clients rather than in-person visits, the HIPAA regulations regarding privacy and security:

    a. Must apply.
    b. Are less stringent.
    c. Can be waived.
    d. Do not apply.

173. **With the disease management model of case management, the case manager focuses on:**
 a. Evidence-based practice to improve outcomes of acute care.
 b. Guiding the client from acute care to post-acute care.
 c. Post-acute services for chronic illness to reduce readmission.
 d. Both caregiving and case management for the client.

174. **If the case manager is part of an interdisciplinary team in which two members of the team have a disagreement regarding client care, the first step to resolving the conflict is to:**
 a. Determine which person has the most reasonable argument.
 b. Encourage the individuals to cooperate.
 c. Remind the individuals that their argument is negatively impacting the team.
 d. Allow both individuals to present their side of issue.

175. **The case manager's primary role in transitions of care is to ensure that:**
 a. The client receives the appropriate level of care and services.
 b. The costs of client care and services don't exceed expectations.
 c. The client is informed about all aspects of client care.
 d. The client understands the need for stepdown or discharge.

176. **In terms of utilization management, an example of underutilization is:**
 a. The average length of stay in the ICU is 8 to 10 days, which is longer than the average.
 b. The hospital lacks an MRI and must transfer clients needing an MRI to another hospital.
 c. A client received an overdose of narcotic and required an extra day of hospitalization.
 d. Routine CBC and urinalysis tests are ordered for all clients in the emergency department.

177. **According to Lewin's force field analysis of change, a driving force would be:**
 a. Hostility.
 b. Lack of equipment.
 c. Insufficient funds.
 d. Competition.

178. **As part of a wellness program, clients with average risk should begin colorectal screening at age:**
 a. 40.
 b. 50.
 c. 60.
 d. 65.

179. **According to the transtheoretical model of change, a client who indicates readiness to change and begins making plans is in the stage of:**
 a. Contemplation.
 b. Action.
 c. Precontemplation.
 d. Preparation.

180. If a 35-year-old client with rheumatoid arthritis has become increasingly withdrawn and socially isolated and states her family and friends don't understand what she is going through, an appropriate intervention is referral to a:

a. Support group.
b. Psychiatrist.
c. Yoga program.
d. Holistic practitioner.

Answer Key and Explanations for Test #2

1. A: While all of these factors are important, reliability is especially important because a reliable vendor usually provides both quality and timely service. Costs may vary somewhat, but the least expensive may not be the best option if equipment is faulty or service is poor. Some community vendors cover a wide area, but this usually poses no problem if they have adequate delivery. Quality is always important, but high quality can sometimes be associated with high costs, so the case manager must determine the level of quality needed. For example, an inexpensive commode chair may be adequate.

2. B: Yes/no questions are the easiest questions to quantify since this type of survey requires only simple addition of two categories, but they provide limited information. **Descriptive/information questions** often provide the most information, but results are difficult to quantify because each individual may answer questions differently. **Multiple-choice questions** must be designed carefully or clients may not find choices that reflect their opinions. These questions are also easy to quantify. **Rating scales** are used primarily to rate satisfaction or to indicate the level of agreement with a statement and—like multiple-choice questions—are easy to quantify.

3. D: The primary purpose of the Caseload Matrix in caseload calculations is to identify variables in various settings affecting caseloads. Elements of the Caseload Matrix that impact the caseload include

- Initial elements: Business environment, market segment, regulatory and legal requirement, clinical practice setting, factors related to individual CM, types/characteristics of CM services, and CM tools, including technology support.
- Comprehensive needs assessment: Clinical factors and client, family, and environmental psychosocial factors.
- CM interventions: CM plan.
- Outcomes: Intermediate, CM, and long term.

4. C: Level 3. The four-point Likert scale is used to assess clients who are at risk of low self-care. The Likert scale has four levels:

- Level 1: A client who is able to attend to normal activities of daily living (ADLs), hygiene, and the environment and has a low risk of failing to adhere to medical regimens/treatments.
- Level 2: A client who has a moderate risk of failing to adhere to medical regimens/treatments and making poor choices.
- Level 3: A client with severe risk of failing to adhere to medical regimens/treatments and making poor choices.
- Level 4: A client whose lack of self-care is extreme and results in self-abuse and neglect.

5. D: People who attempt suicide must be evaluated carefully. Those with a history of previous attempts are especially at risk for suicide. Patients who actually attempt suicide should be hospitalized and assessed for suicide risk after initial treatment. High-risk findings include:

- Violent suicide attempt (knives, gunshots).
- Suicide attempt with low chance of rescue.
- Ongoing psychosis or disordered thinking.
- Ongoing severe depression and feeling of helplessness.
- History of previous suicide attempts.
- Lack of social support system.

6. A: The three-midnight rule for extended Medicare benefit applies to clients transferring to skilled nursing facilities (SNFs). Clients must be under inpatient care for three days (three midnights), but time spent in extended observation in an ED or treatment as an outpatient does not apply. The three-day stay must be justified by care needs. Hospitalization alone does not qualify the client for the extended benefit, as the client must also require daily care at a level appropriate to a SNF.

7. D: InterQual's utilization management tools include **care-planning criteria tools**, which are used to determine if interventions are appropriate and properly sequenced. A **retrospective monitoring tool** evaluates whether surgical and/or medical interventions were appropriate. **Clinical evidence summaries** support recommendations of medical review and encourage the use of evidence-based standards of care. **Level-of-care criteria tools** determine if care is appropriate at different levels, including acute, long-term acute, subacute, skilled nursing facilities, rehabilitation, home health care, chiropractic services, and outpatient rehabilitation services.

8. C: Identifying the need for environmental modifications in a client's home is a role of the case manager under the domain of vocational concepts and strategies. There are **six domains** in which the case manager functions: (1) case finding and intake, (2) provision of CM services, (3) outcomes evaluation/case closure, (4) utilization management, (5) psychosocial and economic issues, and (6) vocational concepts and strategies. Additionally, the case manager has **five roles/responsibilities**: (1) clinical care management, (2) management/leadership, (3) financial and resource management, (4) information management, and (5) professional responsibility.

9. B: Role is a set of expected behaviors and consequences related to a case manager's place in a particular social structure, such as an acute hospital. **Function** refers to a set of tasks that the case manager must complete as part of the role. **Activity** refers to a specific task the case manager performs in order to meet the needs of the role. **Process** refers to a set of activities the case manager carries out to reach a specific goal.

10. C: The CMS Quality Framework for Home and Community Based Services (HCBS) participant safeguards include a process for incident reporting. Other safeguards include risk assessments (taking into consideration a client's right to choose), monitoring of interventions (behavioral/pharmacological), emergency/disaster preparedness, administration of medications, and monitoring of general health condition. Other areas covered by the framework include participation access, client-centered service planning/delivery, capacity of provider, rights and responsibilities, outcomes and client satisfaction, and system preferences.

11. D: The most significant challenge for community-based case managers is the chronically ill because clients with chronic illnesses may have multiple needs, and needs often continue to evolve and increase as the disease progresses. Insurance and Medicare/Medicaid coverage is often inadequate, even though the chronically ill often utilize healthcare resources at a rate higher than others because of their inability to self-manage their conditions. In some cases, the chronically ill may become dependent on healthcare providers, so educating and supporting clients to remain independent are critically important.

12. A: While all of these factors are important to varying degrees, the primary purpose of negotiation in case management practice is to control costs and provide medically necessary services. Cost control was an important factor in developing the case management model, but this must be balanced with providing medically necessary care at the appropriate level. Negotiation can avoid the problems that arise if care is denied. Additionally, negotiation allows participants, including the case manager, to learn new information or learn reasons for decisions or requests.

13. D: While pharmacy assistance plans may vary somewhat from one drug company to another, most set an income limit of less than 200% of the federal poverty level. Many drug companies preclude those with prescription insurance coverage or Medicare D, but some will consider these applicants. Programs usually cover brand name prescription drugs. In most cases, U.S. residency alone is not sufficient; people must be citizens or legal immigrants. Pharmacy assistance programs offer people free drugs or low-cost drugs if the drugs are medically necessary and people cannot afford to purchase them.

14. C: Recent onset under ISD criteria of SI is onset of symptoms within one week. Other criteria include

- **Acute/sudden onset** means symptoms occurred within 24 hours.
- **Recently/newly discovered** means symptoms occurred after one week.
- **Newly discovered** means symptoms occurred during the current episode of sickness.

InterQual's ISD criteria refer to intensity of service (IS), severity of sickness (SS), and discharge screening (DS) regarding the client's stability for discharge. InterQual criteria are used for utilization review and management of clients receiving Medicare and Medicaid benefits.

15. B: Once DME ownership is transferred to a beneficiary, Medicare will pay only for repairs necessary to make the DME serviceable. Medicare no longer pays for routine service or maintenance of DME and now requires that ownership be transferred after specified periods of rental (13 months for most capped DMEs and 36 months for oxygen equipment), after which the cost of rental exceeds the cost of purchase. During the rental period, Medicare also no longer pays for routine service or maintenance, as these are considered covered by the rental fee.

16. A: While there are many factors to consider, the best placement for a 47-year-old male with an IQ of 68 is probably a group home because this is a mild level of intellectual disability, so the client can usually manage self-care with minimal supervision. Group homes are licensed facilities that usually house four to eight clients with similar conditions. Staff members may live in the facility or work in shifts. The quality of group homes may vary widely, so the case manager should be familiar with group homes used for referrals.

17. B: Denial or noncertification may result from extended hospitalization because PT or other services are not available on the weekend. Extended hospitalizations with cause, such as a myocardial infarction, are covered but may require concurrent authorization to notify the payor of changes in condition. A change in policy that takes place after services are rendered should not affect a case, as the effective policy is the one in place at the time of authorization. A client's death should result in termination of benefits rather than denial.

18. D: When a client has comorbidities, the priority in care must be to the condition that is most acute or may be life threatening. While both prostate cancer and pneumonia may be life threatening, pneumonia is the more acute condition and should receive priority. However, this does not mean that other conditions are left untreated, although in some cases aggressive treatment may be delayed. For example, treatment for prostate cancer may be delayed until the pneumonia resolves. Routine treatment for hypertension and Type 1 diabetes may continue, but educating the client about disease management may be postponed.

19. B: According to the Agency for Healthcare Research and Quality (AHRQ) data, the average length of stay in a hospital after a complete knee replacement is about 4 days (3.9), after which most clients transfer to a SNF or rehabilitation center for continued therapy. Reducing LOS is a major factor in reducing costs and complications, as prolonged hospitalization is more likely to result in infection. Stays beyond the average for a particular condition may result in denial of services or increased scrutiny to determine the cause.

20. C: A client becomes an inpatient only after the doctor changes the order to have the client admitted as an inpatient. People receiving outpatient/ambulatory surgery may in some cases stay overnight, especially if their surgery was performed late in the day or if they prolonged observation. Even with an overnight stay, people are still considered outpatients. The distinction is important because the basis for payment differs for inpatient services and outpatient services.

21. C: National indicators for emergency department crowding include:

- **Diversions:** Number of hours the ED is unable to accept clients because it has reached capacity, requiring diversion of clients to other facilities.
- **Boarding:** Number of clients who must remain in the ED awaiting admission because the hospital has no beds available or no staff available to prepare rooms or facilitate transfer.
- **Clients are leaving the ED after triage:** If there is a substantial delay in time between triage and evaluation, some clients leave the ED for various reasons, such as impatience, transportation needs, or family responsibilities. Some seek medical care elsewhere.

22. A: The case manager in an admitting department serves essentially as a gatekeeper to determine if admission to acute care is necessary or if a lower level of care is indicated. The case manager is responsible for acquiring preauthorization of care or certifications as needed. Additionally, the case manager communicates information about the client and client's condition to the insurance company/payor to support a request for authorization or to discuss the need for other care.

23. C: Because of perceived excess costs associated with occupational, physical, and speech therapy, careful documentation must include realistic and measurable goals as well as a physician's order for therapy and evidence that therapy was provided by or supervised by a licensed therapist who conducted a thorough evaluation and developed a plan of care that included frequency and duration of treatment. Documentation must also indicate that the therapy was medically necessary. The same documentation requirements apply to skilled nursing facilities.

24. B: An electronic alarmed medication delivery device can hold up to 30 days' supply of medications and can be set to deliver the medications at a particular time or times each day, with an alarm sounding when the medication cup is full. While someone may need to fill the device one or two times monthly, this is more cost effective than hiring someone daily to give medications and allows the client to remain more independent in care.

25. C: The Older Americans Act (OAA) provides a wide range of home and community services for older adults as well as respite services for family caregivers for older adults and children with special needs. OAA programs include support of senior centers, nutrition services, respite programs, and long-term care planning. The OAA also supports health, prevention, and wellness programs that include Alzheimer's disease, diabetes, HIV/AIDS, and self-management of chronic disease as well as the Healthy People 2030 initiative. The OAA is also involved with protection of elder rights through legal assistance, pension counseling and information services, and ombudsman programs.

26. A: Initial symptom management of shortness of breath in a palliative care client includes elevating the head and aiming a fan toward the person's face to circulate air. Up to 80% of palliative care clients may experience some degree of dyspnea, which can usually be managed conservatively. If dyspnea is severe, as may occur with lung disease, an opioid (usually morphine) or sedative (benzodiazepines) may be indicated. Corticosteroids are used for specific cases, such as those with superior vena cava syndrome. Oxygen by facemask may relieve dyspnea for some patients. Bronchodilators are indicated if shortness of breath is associated with bronchospasm.

27. B: Change theory:

- **Motivation to change (unfreezing):** Dissatisfaction occurs when goals are not met, but as previous beliefs are brought into question, survival anxiety occurs. Sometimes learning anxiety about having to learn different strategies causes resistance that can lead to denial, blaming others, and trying to maneuver or bargain without real change.
- **Desire to change (unfrozen):** Dissatisfaction is strong enough to override defensive actions, and desire to change is strong but must be coupled with identification of needed changes.
- **Development of permanent change (refreezing):** New behavior becomes habitual, often requiring a change in perceptions of self and establishment of new relationships.

28. A: Pastoral counseling provides a bridge between religion and therapy, with members of the clergy trained as mental health professionals, usually with a master's degree or doctorate. A client who may be reluctant to see a psychologist may be more receptive to one that engages spirituality and prayer as part of therapy. Pastoral counselors serve those with mental health disorders and substance abuse disorders as well as providing family and couples therapy. They may also promote wellness/spirituality programs.

29. D: While state programs for long-term care may vary, in general, all states provide for those with low income requiring long-term care because of complex illnesses that need extensive care or multiple physical or mental problems that preclude clients' caring for themselves. Most state programs have strict financial guidelines and limit the amount of savings and/or property a person can own, and the application process can take up to three months, so the case manager should explore this option early.

30. C: To facilitate the continuum of care after a client is discharged from an acute hospital, the case manager should establish ongoing relationships with staff and administrators of skilled nursing facilities, home health agencies, subacute and rehabilitation facilities, as well as assisted living facilities because the services they provide may be critical to allow the client to safely be discharged. Establishing relationships with physician's staff, hospital administrators, and HMO clinicians is usually more important for preadmission issues.

31. A: Health Status Survey (SF-36 or SF-12) is a tool that provides a client's self-assessment of functional health and quality-of-life issues. The **Patient Health Questionnaire** (PHQ) is used to screen patients and monitor conditions related to mental health disorders, such as depression and anxiety and substance abuse. The **Post Deployment Clinical Assessment Tool (PDCAT)** is used to screen returning military for mental health and substance abuse problems related to deployment, including PTSD, depression, anxiety, and alcoholism. The **Barthel Index** assesses the functional ability of older adults in relation to activities of daily living.

32. D: Support groups help members who share a common problem, such as the stress of caregiving, learn to cope. **Education groups** provide information to group members about specific issues, such as managing medication or disease. **Self-help groups** are usually informal groups without professional leaders intended for members who share a common experience, such as Alcoholics Anonymous. **Psychotherapy groups** teach members about their behavior and methods to change by interacting with others.

33. C: The **Brain Trauma Foundation (BTF)** has taken an active role in preventing concussions and provides checklists and videos and other information. The BTF also provides information about comas and guidelines for care of traumatic brain injury (TBI). The **American College of Sports Medicine** is intended for professionals and students involved in sports medicine and exercise, providing research and information about effective techniques. The **American Association of Physical Medicine and Rehabilitation** is a medical society for physicians engaged in physical medicine and rehabilitation. The **Orthopedic Research Society** promotes multidisciplinary collaborations in orthopedic care and dissemination of current research.

34. B: The primary purpose of a health coach is to guide clients to discuss concerns regarding recovery, including obstacles and the need for support. The health coach specifically avoids prescribing treatment, advising, and counseling because the focus remains on the client and helping the client develop the motivation to change and reach goals. Health coaching was initially used to help people recover from substance abuse, but it is now also used to help people cope with chronic illnesses and adopt a healthier lifestyle.

35. C: Clients who resort to eating only candy and snack foods usually do so because these foods are easy to obtain and require no preparation, so the best intervention is home delivery of meals, such as Meals on Wheels programs. While an occupational therapist may help the man learn ways to prepare meals with less exertion and nutritional counseling may help the client understand the need to eat better meals, home delivery of meals is the most direct and simple intervention. Since the man is managing other aspects of care, he does not yet require assisted living.

36. B: The first step in crisis intervention is a thorough evaluation and assessment of the problem and the triggering event as well as assessment of risks, such as suicide. A plan should be devised in collaboration with the individual, taking resources into consideration. Steps in intervention include:

- Helping the individual to gain understanding about the cause of the crisis.
- Encouraging the individual to freely express thoughts and feelings.
- Teaching the individual different coping mechanisms and adaptive behaviors.
- Encouraging social interaction.

37. B: Depression often goes undiagnosed, so screening for at-risk individuals should be done routinely. Depression is associated with conditions that decrease quality of life, such as heart disease, neuromuscular diseases, arthritis, cancer, diabetes, Huntington's disease, stroke, and diabetes. Some drugs may also precipitate depression: diuretics, Parkinson's drugs, estrogen, corticosteroids, cimetidine, hydralazine, propranolol, digitalis, and indomethacin. Patients experience changes in mood, sadness, loss of interest in usual activities, increased fatigues, changes in appetite and fluctuations in weight, anxiety, and sleep disturbance.

38. A: Problem solving involves actively searching for a way to reduce stress and cope. **Avoidance** means to avoid stressors or reduce their impact if possible. **Physical activity** can often increase feelings of well-being and allow people to cope more effectively. **Spirituality** can involve attending religious services or engaging in religious or spiritual endeavors to provide emotional support and a positive outlook. Those with ineffective coping skills may express anxiety, anger, and agitation (which may interfere with decision making) and may develop depression and physical ailments, such as anorexia, weight loss, nausea, urinary and bowel problems, and sleep disturbance.

39. D: According to the Dying Person's Bill of Rights, every patient has a right to hope and to participate in religious/spiritual experiences, so the correct response is "What can I do to help?" The case manager should not state that the healing is unrealistic or put the burden on the patient with "If you believe . . ." Patients have a right to seek spiritual guidance and/or healing without a doctor's permission. Traditional Hmong families may shun Western medicine and rely solely on healers, while Christian Hmong may rely only on Western medicine. However, many Hmong people straddle both the traditional and Western worlds.

40. A: Dual diagnosis is a combined substance abuse and a mental health disorder. The initial treatment usually involves detoxification to stop the use of drugs so that the mental health condition can be more accurately evaluated. This is followed by rehabilitation, such as a drug recovery program, and mental health treatment, which can include medications [such as selective serotonin reuptake inhibitors (SSRIs) or psychotropics] or therapy, including group and cognitive-behavioral therapy. In some cases, people abuse drugs to self-treat mental illnesses, but in other cases, the mental illnesses result from drug abuse.

41. A: Health literacy primarily requires basic reading, numerical, comprehension, and communication skills. Clients should be able to read and understand prescription labels and warnings, insurance forms, and consent forms. They should be able to do basic math to calculate doses when necessary, and they should be able to comprehend basic information about disease and self-management. They need the ability to communicate their concerns and needs and to comprehend instructions and health information. Motivation alone is not enough, but an above-average intellectual ability is not necessary.

42. D: Bereavement is the time period of mourning. This time period varies but may extend to a year or even longer. **Grief** is a normal response to loss while **mourning** is the public expression of grief. There are three types of grief: acute, anticipatory, and chronic. **Chronic grief** poses a serious risk to people and should be treated as depression, with antidepressants, psychological evaluation, and counselling. **Depression** is characterized by changes in mood and feelings of sadness.

43. C: One indication of financial abuse is the disappearance of items from the home. Family, friends, or caregivers may begin taking one or two items at a time, assuming the person will not notice. Other types of financial abuse include:

- Outright stealing of property or persuading patients to give away possessions.
- Forcing patients to sign away property.
- Emptying bank and savings accounts.
- Using stolen credit cards.
- Convincing the person to invest money in fraudulent schemes.
- Taking money for home renovations that are not done.

Indications of financial abuse may be unpaid bills, unusual activity at ATMs, and inadequate funds to meet needs.

44. B: The case manager should outline objectives of a call prior to telephoning a client to review status. This helps to maintain focus and ensures that all necessary topics are covered. Preparing a script in advance is not necessary and may seem "faked" to the client. The case manager should be prepared to guide the conversation and answer potential questions the client may have. It is not necessary to mail a notification, but the case manager should, if possible, advise the client that follow-up may be done by phone as clients may be reluctant to divulge personal information over the phone.

45. D: The CMSA standard of Facilitation, Coordination, and Collaboration can be demonstrated by the use of mediation and/or negotiation to facilitate communication. The CMSA Standards of Practice (2016) comprise 15 standards: client selection (includes use of screening for high-risk clients); client assessment; problem/opportunity identification; planning; outcomes; monitoring (includes documentation of ongoing efforts at collaboration); termination of CM services (includes documentation of termination of care); facilitation, coordination, and collaboration; qualifications; legal; ethics, advocacy, cultural competency, resource management/stewardship; and research/research utilization.

46. B: The case manager should immediately place the client on a second shelter waiting list to increase the chance for placement, even though the client may prefer a different shelter. Discharging a client into the streets poses an ethical dilemma, and if no placement can be found, then Social Services may be able to provide some alternatives. The decision about calling daily depends on the individual shelter and the relationship the case manager has with the shelter administration. Transferring to a level of care that is higher than needed is not a viable option even with Medicaid, and the client is indigent and uninsured.

47. B: Bloodshot eyes, sniffing repeatedly, altered sleeping habits, and marked weight loss are typical signs of cocaine use. Cocaine depresses the appetite, so a sudden drop in weight may be one of the first signs. Because cocaine is often snorted, it can damage the septum and mucous membranes of the nose, causing the nose to run constantly. Clients may go without sleep for long periods followed by long periods of sleeping. Eyes become bloodshot from irritation.

48. D: A Glasgow coma score of 10 (more than 8) suggests the potential for rehabilitation. A score of 3 to 8 indicates coma, while a score of 9 to 12 indicates severe head injury and 13 to 15 indicates mild head injury. The Glasgow Coma Scale (GCS) measures the depth and duration of coma or impaired consciousness and is used for postoperative assessment. The GCS measures three parameters: best eye response, best verbal response, and best motor response, with a total possible score that ranges from 3 to 15.

49. D: An assisted living/custodial care facility is the appropriate placement for a client who has slight dementia but is otherwise medically stable and can ambulate and toilet independently. Unlicensed staff may assist patients to take routine medications and perform simple dry dressing changes, although a home health nurse may be necessary if care is more complex. Clients may have home oxygen but should not require tracheal suctioning. Assisted living facilities are not usually appropriate for clients in need of rehabilitation or those who are more confused or disoriented because of safety concerns.

50. D: Unskilled care includes taking and reporting routine vital signs, assisting clients to take medications, assisting with personal care (bathing, applying lotions and creams, changing simple dressings), preparing meals, assisting with feeding, emptying drainage bags and measuring drainage, assisting with colostomy and ileostomy care, administering medical gases (after client has stabilized), providing chest physiotherapy, assisting with stable tracheostomy care, and supervising exercises prescribed by a therapist as well as performing simple range-of-motion (active and passive) exercises, and utilizing or helping clients use assistive devices.

51. B: A client or parent's refusal of care may be overridden in only a few instances, including when the client is mentally incompetent to make decisions, although advance directives completed prior to onset of dementia may remain valid. Other factors that may result in overriding refusal of care include life-threatening conditions for minor children and conditions that put the general public at risk, such as with those who refuse treatment for resistive forms of tuberculosis or other highly communicable diseases.

52. A: Poverty is a risk factor for malnutrition as people may be unable to purchase nutritious foods. Other risk factors include recent weight gain or loss of 10 pounds or more and ill-fitting dentures, lack of teeth, tooth abscesses, and dental caries. Those with a history of eating disorders (bulimia, anorexia) are at risk as well as those with acute or chronic illnesses. People who live alone or are socially isolated may experience loss of appetite. Disabilities may interfere with the ability to purchase and/or prepare foods.

53. C: Clients who experience an unintentional overdose should be referred for a psychosocial evaluation because the overdose may result from lack of knowledge, inability to read instructions, or polydrug use. Other indications include intentional overdoses, substance abuse (illegal or prescription drugs, alcohol), eating disorders (anorexia, bulimia), chronic mental illness, and dementia. In some cases, referrals are indicated based on behavior, such as repeated hospitalizations, noncompliance with treatment regimen, and aggressive or uncooperative behavior. Homelessness, heart disease, and limited financial sources do not necessarily indicate a need for psychosocial evaluation.

54. B: Breach is the legal element of negligence that refers to a failure to carry out duties in accordance with accepted and usual standards of practice. **Duty** is a legal responsibility or obligation that relates to a relationship (such as parent to protect his/her child) or statute (such as the requirement for a case manager to report child abuse). **Causation** is the direct proof that a breach of duty resulted in harm. **Harm** is the injury that results from a breach of duty.

55. A: Because **fine motor impairment** interferes with a person's ability to use the hands, a job accommodation might include a speech recognition program for computer access as well as alternative methods to answer the phone and adaptive writing materials, ergonomic tools, page turners, grip devices, book holders, arm supports, and modified keyboards. Those with **gross motor impairment** may require modification in the workstation, stand/lean stools, rolling safety ladders, desktop Lazy Susans, and carts to transport materials.

56. D: The client most likely to need and benefit from case management is the 72-year-old woman with a postoperative wound infection after hip replacement because the infection may result in both an extended stay in the acute hospital as well as in a SNF and increased need for medications and other treatments. If osteomyelitis develops, then chronic care may be necessary. People with uncomplicated procedures, such as appendectomy and TURP, usually do not need case management. The diabetic's insulin reaction probably resulted from the vomiting and diarrhea and will resolve with treatment.

57. C: When converting to an interoperable healthcare delivery system, the most important aspect to consider is the need for extensive training for all staff at all levels because all procedures that are currently paper related must be modified and converted to a digital format. Standard terminology may need to be established or modified. Staff must be trained to input information in the electronic system as well as to retrieve information, and safeguards must be built into the system to prevent violations of confidentiality. Information retrievable over the Internet must be encrypted.

58. B: The medical home model is a client-centered model of care in which a primary care physician manages, facilitates, and coordinates all levels of client care, including care provided by specialists. The leader (physician) usually receives some type of additional payment for providing the service. Clients may be assigned to a medical home or may, in some cases, choose one. The goal is to decrease the fragmented and uncoordinated care that many clients receive in order to improve client outcomes.

59. D: Work hardening is using real tasks or simulated work-related tasks and progressive exercises to strengthen and condition a person to return to the workplace. **Work adjustment** is assessing work behavior to determine behaviors that are appropriate and inappropriate and then providing support to increase appropriate behaviors and improve job skills. **Transitional employment** is the noncompetitive employment placement utilized with job coaching. **Job coaching** is placing a person in a position and using a job specialist to train the employee to do specific job-related tasks and to learn the necessary interpersonal skills needed for the job.

60. A: Subacute and rehabilitation facilities usually provide IV care that can include infusion pumps and multiple IV medications. These facilities also provide ongoing monitoring by RNs and manage complex drug regimens. They may also care for people on respirations or those requiring tracheal suctions and can provide tube care for gastrostomy and jejunostomy, T-tubes, and catheters as well as colostomy and ileostomy care. Complex wound care is available as well as at least two types of rehabilitation therapy (speech, physical therapy, occupational therapy).

61. C: Inconsistencies in social, medical, and functional data are not uncommon, so the case manager should first consult with the source of inconsistent data to try to determine the reason for the inconsistency. In some cases, the inconsistency may result from error or misstatements. In other cases, the client's condition may have changed from one assessment to another. The client usually serves as the primary source of information, but other sources can include family, friends, employers, physicians, other healthcare providers (such as home health nurses and physical therapists), and medical records.

62. B: Intermediate care provides people with moderate assistance in activities of daily living and periodic nursing supervision for some activities, such as assistance with ambulation, grooming, and medications. Insurance companies usually do not pay for this level. **Custodial care/assisted living** provides people with assistance performing basic ADLs, such as dressing and bathing. Insurance companies do not pay for this level. **Skilled nursing** provides maximal assistance with ADLs and the need for daily supervision/care by a licensed professional. Insurance companies usually pay for this level. **Acute care** can include hospitals, rehabilitation services, inpatient rehabilitation centers, and transitional hospitals. Insurance companies should pay for this level.

63. C: For clients who receive oxygen at >4L/min, blood gases must be drawn at 4L/min. Testing must be done within two days of discharge to home or while the client is in a "chronic stable state." Other qualifying criteria include:

- Blood gases drawn on room air (if requires oxygen <4L/min).
- PO_2 ≤55 with arterial saturation ≤88%.
- PO_2 56 to 59 with arterial saturation ≤89% with dependent edema, P-pulmonale, or Hct >56%. (Requires retesting between days 61 and 90 of oxygen therapy.)
- Documentation must include diagnosis of severe lung disease and indication that alternative treatments were ineffective.

64. C: When a person is sitting and working on a computer, the elbows should be bent at a 90-degree angle and wrists held straight. The seat of the chair should be adjusted so that the person's feet are flat on the floor (or on a foot stool if the person is short) and the knees also bent at a 90-degree angle. The chair should provide support in the lower back, and the angle of the back of the chair to the seat should be 90 degrees.

65. B: Assistive devices include shower chairs, handrails, adaptive kitchen equipment, ostomy and wound care supplies. **Mobility aids** include crutches, canes, walkers, wheelchairs, and scooters. **High-technology equipment** includes apnea/sleep monitors, ventilators, parenteral/enteral nutrition, infusion pumps, and specialized electronic/computerized equipment for quadriplegia/paraplegia. **Cognitive aids** include devices that help those with memory or other mental difficulties. Durable medical equipment must be approved, and Medicare regulations require the equipment be purchased from a Medicare-participating supplier.

66. A: Underutilization may result from delays in performing necessary diagnostic procedures. Other causes of underutilization include insurance denial of services, lack of adequate monitoring of client's response to treatment, complications (such as pressure sores), and transfers to the wrong level of care. **Overutilization** may result from client's insistence on expensive procedures, client's being in a teaching hospital, physician's concern about liability (defensive medicine), duplicate testing, frequency of testing, choice of medication, and route of administration.

67. C: Indemnity plans offer the most flexibility because they do not have provider lists or other restrictions commonly found in managed care. Clients are usually free to see whatever physician they want, although some plans require prehospital certification. Additionally, indemnity plans are often more expensive and may have varying deductibles (up to $5000), and plans usually only pay a percentage of costs (usually 80%) so out-of-pocket expenses to the client are often higher. Plans may have limits (duration or dollar amounts) on some types of care, such as drug treatment programs.

68. D: A **prospective or preadmission review** takes place prior to admission and determines whether admission to a facility is justified and necessary and will be authorized by the insurance company, although the physician may override the insurance company. A **concurrent review** occurs during care to determine if care is appropriate. A **retrospective review** occurs after discharge and determines if payment will be authorized or denied. This is less common since many insurance companies now require preauthorization for services. A **telephonic review** is usually concurrent but is conducted by phone rather than in person.

69. B: As a client advocate, the case manager's primary responsibility when conflicts arise over coverage is to the client, ensuring that the client's healthcare needs are met and that the client has information necessary for self-advocacy. This may include educating the client to clients' rights and providing information about appeals processes although the case manager usually does not assist directly with appeals. When a case manager is employed directly by a payor or care provider, a conflict of interest may occur if the case manager feels pressured to support the employer.

70. A: Process measures determine if correct action, such as cervical cancer screening and administration of antibiotics within six hours for pneumonia, were completed. **Outcomes measures** evaluate the success of care and include measures of falls, surgical site infections, blood pressure control, 30-day mortality rates for MI, and number of adults evaluated for weight. **Patient experience measures** use surveys to determine clients' views on the care they have received. **Structural measures** provide information about conditions such as nursing care hours, e-prescribing, and number of medical homes. **Composite measures** combine information to provide an overview, including mortality rates for different conditions and pediatric safety.

71. D: The **Instrumental Activities of Daily Living** (IADL) tool assesses financial ability (ability to pay bills, budget, and keep track of finances), telephone use, shopping, food preparation, housekeeping, laundry, transportation availability (ability to drive or use public transportation), and medications (ability to manage prescriptions and take medications). The **Barthel Index of Activities of Daily Living** assesses 10 categories, usually including bathing, toileting, ascending or descending stairs, feeding, mobility, personal grooming, urinary and fecal control, transferring, and ambulatory/wheelchair status.

72. A: Community variances include insurance delays, unavailability of DME, beds in SNF, and beds in shelters, regional disasters, and delay in arrival of child protective services. **Practitioner variances** include late orders, inaccessibility to physician or specialist, orders for inappropriate levels of care, early or late physician visits, incompetent care, delayed review of tests, inappropriate medical equipment, and failure to receive authorization. **Institution/systems** variances include delay in transcribing orders and providing services, equipment malfunction or lack of necessary equipment, and unnecessary 72-hour hospitalization before transfer. **Client/family variances** include unsafe or unsupportive family environment, medical complications, no clothes or needed supplies, indecision, and knowledge deficit.

73. C: An environmental assessment includes not only specific rooms in the home but also general needs and includes evaluations of:

- Environmental hazards: Piles of paper or junk, loose carpets, cluttered pathways.
- Lighting: Adequate for reading in all rooms and stairways.
- Heat and air-conditioning: Adequate for environment to control heat and cold.
- Sanitation: Rotting food, infestations of cockroaches or rodents.
- Animal care: Pets should have access to food, water, toileting, and veterinary care.
- Smoke/chemicals in the environment: Second-hand smoke or cleaning chemicals.

74. B: The learner outcome for teaching a client about insulin reaction should relate directly to that goal: List and describe the symptoms of insulin reaction. While all of the other things (different types of insulin, foods high in carbohydrates, and the difference between Type 1 and Type 2 diabetes) are important, they don't relate to the topic and should not be the learner outcome for this activity. In some cases, one class or session may cover multiple topics with multiple outcomes, but a client may be overwhelmed by too much information.

75. A: Case management is people-oriented because the focus is on all the people involved in client care, including the client, to provide necessary services in a coordinated and collaborative manner. While cost-containment and nursing considerations are aspects of case management, they are not primary. **Managed care**, which focuses on people's benefits, such as insurance coverage, is systems-oriented and is more economically focused on efforts to contain costs while providing good client care. Managed care is also concerned with the regulations affecting delivery of care.

76. B: Because women were routinely being discharged within 24 hours after labor and delivery of an infant in the 1980s and 1990s and insurance companies were denying longer care, Congress enacted the Newborns' and Mothers' Health Protection Act (1996) to ensure that mothers and infants could remain in the hospital for longer periods. This act mandated stays of 48 hours after uncomplicated birth and 96 hours after Caesarean birth unless a mother waives this requirement and chooses to be discharged earlier.

77. B: Eligibility for CM certification requires six conditions: (1) The applicant is licensed or certified to practice independently. (2) Employment experience has to be completed before application process and (3) must focus on case management ≥30% of the time. (4) Applicant performs all eight essential activities and (5) performs work within at least five of six core components. (6) Within each of these components, the applicant performs all eight essential activities, provides services extending through the continuum of care, interacts with other healthcare providers, and is primarily responsible for managing client's needs.

78. D: For those who are eligible, Medicare may cover home health care to provide occupational therapy, speech therapy, and physical therapy as well as skilled nursing services on an intermittent basis (less than seven days weekly or eight hours daily). Those receiving skilled care may also receive services of a home health aide to assist with personal care. Home delivery of meals, 24-hour care, and homemaker or aide services alone are not covered by Medicare.

79. C: Integrative. A number of different **types of outcomes data** must be considered:

- **Integrative**: This includes measures of mortality, longevity, and cost-effectiveness.
- **Clinical**: This includes symptoms, diagnoses, staging of disease and those indicators of individual health.
- **Physiological**: This includes measures of physical abnormalities, loss of function, and activities of daily living.
- **Psychosocial**: This includes feelings, perceptions, beliefs, functional impairment, and role performance.
- **Perception**: This includes customer perceptions, evaluations, and satisfaction.
- **Organization-wide clinical**: This includes readmissions, adverse reactions, and deaths.

80. B: The primary focus of Workers' Compensation, a type of insurance, is to return people to work as quickly and safely as possible. Workers' Compensation is intended for those who are injured on the job or whose health is impaired because of their jobs. Workers' Compensation provides three different types of benefits: cash to replace lost wages, reimbursement for medical costs associated with the injury, and death benefits to survivors. Workers' Compensation laws may vary somewhat from one state to another.

81. C: A **case mix group** (CMG) is a classification system based on clinical characteristics of clients in rehabilitation care settings. The **resource utilization group** (RUG) is a classification system based on utilization of resources with reimbursement tied to RUG level for skilled nursing facilities. The **Outcome and Assessment Information Set** (OASIS) is a data set used by home health agencies (HHA) to measure outcomes and risk factors within a specified time frame. A **minimum data set** (MDS) contains elements to review for a comprehensive assessment of client function.

82. A: For questions about coverage for self-funded, employer-sponsored health plans, the case manager should contact the benefits manager for the plan. Employers usually contract with consultants or companies that specialize in benefits management, and this information should be on the insurance card. In many cases, employers also have stop-loss policies so that if costs exceed a specified amount (such as $50,000) then the stop-loss insurance covers the claims. In this case, the case manager may be referred to a different benefits manager.

83. B: The primary purpose of pharmacy benefit (PB) management is to reduce the cost of drugs. The PB manager serves as a third-party administrator for drug prescription plans. The PBM negotiates lower prices, encourages lower cost bulk mail delivery (usually providing a 90-day supply of drugs), encourages the use of generic drugs (usually by reducing the price compared to brand-name drugs), provides a formulary for clients, and promotes drug safety through the use of electronic prescriptions to prevent drug errors.

84. D: FIM™ scores range from 18 (total dependence) to 126 (total independence), and a score of 63 comprised of 3 or 4 in each of 18 categories suggests the need for minimal to moderate contact assistance. The client will require an aide to assist with ambulation and other activities. Lower FIM scores on admission correlate with longer need for inpatient rehabilitation. FIM scores are included as part of the Inpatient Rehabilitation Facility Client Assessment Instrument required by Medicare for reimbursement for care.

85. D: The first step in a cultural assessment is to establish trust by respecting ethnic and cultural values and traditions, being a good listener, and making careful observations. Because a cultural assessment is part of an overall evaluation, asking permission or explaining the purpose of the cultural assessment specifically is usually not necessary. In some cultures, taking notes while talking is considered rude, so the nurse should explain the purpose and take brief notes, keeping the focus on the client and family instead of the paperwork.

86. B: Intensive case management for assertive community treatment is a form of community-monitored medical care focused on providing support for those with serious mental health issues and the inability to function independently in the community without a multifaceted approach because of difficulties with employment, personal relationships, financial management, and physical health. An interdisciplinary team, which many include occupational therapists, vocational trainers, counselors, psychiatrists, nurses, support services, and peer counselors, provides intensive and proactive support, assisting the client to avoid crisis situations or deal successfully with them.

87. A: Palliative care can begin when a client is diagnosed with a life-threatening disease, such as advanced cancer or amyotrophic lateral sclerosis (ALS). In some cases, those with serious chronic diseases, such as chronic obstructive pulmonary disease (COPD) may be referred for palliative care even though death does not appear imminent. A client request alone for palliative care is not adequate unless the client has an appropriate diagnosis. Palliative care may be simply supportive in the early stages but intensifies as a client's condition deteriorates.

88. A: Steps to conflict resolution include:

- First, allow both sides to present their side of conflict without bias, maintaining a focus on opinions rather than individuals.
- Encourage cooperation through negotiation and compromise.
- Maintain focus, providing guidance to keep the discussions on track and avoid arguments.
- Evaluate the need for renegotiation, formal resolution process, or third-party intervention.

The best time for conflict resolution is when differences emerge but before open conflict and hardening of positions occur. The nurse must pay close attention to the people and problems involved, listen carefully, and reassure those involved that their points of view are understood.

89. B: Usual COBRA coverage for an employee who was voluntarily or involuntarily terminated (unless for gross misconduct) or had reduction in hours of employment is 18 months if meeting eligibility requirements, which include prior enrollment in the insurance plan that remains in effect for active employees. If disability occurs during the 18 months and is supported by a ruling from the SSA, then coverage may be extended an additional 11 months at up to 150% of premium cost. Divorced spouses and dependent children may have benefits extended to 36 months.

90. C: The primary criterion for referral to a hospice program is the probability that death will occur within six months. Generally, hospice programs require a DNR order and a diagnosis of a life-threatening disease, but those alone are not sufficient, as those with longer life expectancies should be referred to palliative care programs instead. Severe intractable pain may be one problem hospice addresses, but pain can occur in clients who do not have a life-threatening disease.

91. D: Hard savings, such as changing the length of stay, are costs that are specifically saved or avoided based on interventions of the case manager. Hard savings may also derive from changes in level of care, change to a preferred provider organization (PPO), negotiations for price saving, changes in frequency or duration of services, and identifying unauthorized charges. **Soft savings** are potential savings that cannot be directly attributed to the action of the case manager. These can include preventive measures that avoid hospital readmissions as well as avoiding home health care, and preventing medical errors.

92. A: A child life specialist has a broad knowledge of child development and expertise in developmental assessments, working with families, preparing children for painful or unpleasant procedures, and therapeutic play and can address the unique needs, both physical and emotional, of children of all ages. Additionally, child life specialists can serve as resources for other healthcare providers and families to help them gain more knowledge about the needs and care of children. Child life specialists are trained in stress-reduction techniques to reduce anxiety in children and their families.

93. B: Gross negligence. Negligence indicates that *proper care* has not been provided, based on established standards. *Reasonable care* uses rationale for decision making in relation to providing care. Types of negligence include:

- **Negligent conduct** indicates that an individual failed to provide reasonable care or to protect/assist another, based on standards and expertise.
- **Gross negligence** is willfully providing inadequate care while disregarding the safety and security of another.
- **Contributory negligence** involves the injured party contributing to his/her own harm.
- **Comparative negligence** attempts to determine what percentage amount of negligence is attributed to each individual involved.

94. B: The hospital must develop a discharge plan if ordered to by a physician. There is no other option: Simplified plans or substituting general information materials is not acceptable. The discharge planning process must be applied to all clients and must include identifying clients in need of the plan, completing a discharge planning evaluation that includes whether the client is expected to need posthospital services. This discharge planning evaluation must be included in the client's medical record and discussed with the client.

95. C: The legal document that designates someone to make decisions regarding medical and end-of-life care if a client is mentally incompetent is a durable power of attorney. This is a type of advance directive, which can include living wills or specific requests of the client regarding treatment. A do-not-resuscitate order indicates that the client does not want resuscitative treatment for a terminal illness or condition. A general power of attorney allows a designated person to make decisions for a person over broader areas, including financial.

96. C: Justice is the ethical principle that relates to the distribution of the limited resources of healthcare benefits to the members of society. These resources must be distributed fairly. This issue may arise if there is only one bed left and two clients. Justice comes into play in deciding which client should stay and which should be transported or otherwise cared for. The decision should be made according to what is best or most just for the clients and not colored by personal bias.

97. C: Family Systems Theory states that members of a family have different roles and behavioral patterns, so a change in one person's behavior will affect the others in the family. The **Health Belief Model** predicts health behavior with the understanding that people take a health action to avoid negative consequences if the person expects that the negative outcome can be avoided and that he/she is able to do the action. The **Theory of Reasoned Action** states the actions people take voluntarily can be predicted according to their personal attitude toward the action and their perception of how others will view their doing the action. The **Theory of Planned Behavior** evolved from the Theory of Reasoned Action when studies showed behavioral intention does not necessarily result in action.

98. A: Kolb's model of experiential learning is based on acquiring knowledge through grasping experience and transforming that experience into knowledge through cognitive processes and perception. Experience may be transformed into knowledge through abstract conceptualizing (analyzing, thinking), observation of others, or actively experimenting. This model stresses that the

95

individual makes choices between the concrete and the abstract, and this is reflected in learning styles:

- Diverging: Concrete experience and reflective observation.
- Assimilating: Abstract conceptualization and reflective observation.
- Converging: Abstract conceptualization and active experimentation.
- Accommodating: Concrete experience and reflective observation.

99. A: "The law doesn't allow me to give out any information about clients in order to protect their privacy and safety" is accurate and appropriate. The Health Insurance Portability and Accountability Act (HIPAA) addresses the privacy of health information. Psychiatric/mental health nurses must not release any information or documentation about a client's condition or treatment without consent. Personal information about the client is considered protected health information (PHI), and it includes any identifying or personal information about the client, such as health history, condition, or treatments in any form, and any documentation. Failure to comply with HIPAA regulations can make a nurse liable for legal action.

100. D: Targeted. **Primary prevention** strategies include

- **Targeted:** Aimed at a select group or subgroup with perceived risk. Strategies may include encouraging physicians to intervene with brief advice, such as advising all adolescents about the dangers of substance abuse.
- **Universal:** Aimed at the entire population, nonspecific. These strategies may include mass-marketing procedures, such as multimedia antidrug campaigns aimed at the general public.
- **Indicated:** Aimed at individuals at high risk, such as adolescents in environments with heavy drug use.
- **Secondary prevention:** Includes efforts to prevent further drug abuse, such as Narcotics Anonymous.

101. A: A **cost/benefit analysis** uses average cost of an event and the cost of intervention to demonstrate savings. A **cost-effective analysis** measures the effectiveness of an intervention rather than the monetary savings. **Efficacy studies** may compare a series of cost/benefit analyses to determine the intervention with the best cost/benefit. They may also be used for process or product evaluation. **Cost/utility analysis** (CUA) is essentially a subtype of cost-effective analysis, but it is more complex and the results are more difficult to quantify and use to justify expense because cost/utility analysis measures the benefit to society in general, such as decreasing teen pregnancy.

102. B: Tracer methodology looks at the continuum of care a client receives from admission to post discharge. A client is selected to be "traced," and the medical record serves as a guide. Tracer methodology uses the experience of this client to evaluate the processes in place through documents and interviews. **Root cause analysis (RCA)** is a retrospective attempt to determine the cause of an event, often a sentinel event such as an unexpected death or a cluster of events. Root cause analysis involves interviews, observations, and review of medical records. **Family and staff surveys** may provide helpful but may contain less detailed information.

103. B: The case manager should not disclose personal information, such as impending divorce, because this establishes a social relationship that interferes with the professional role of the nurse. Small tokens of appreciation that can be shared with other staff, such as a box of chocolates, are usually acceptable (depending upon the policy of the institution), but almost any other gifts (jewelry, money, clothes) should be declined. Assisting a client to place a phone call is not a boundary issue. Touching should be used with care, such as touching a hand or shoulder. Hugging may be misconstrued.

104. D: While all of these characteristics are important for team members, central to collaboration is the willingness to compromise. In addition, members must be able to communicate clearly, which encompasses assertiveness, patience, and empathy. Teams should identify specific challenges and problems and then focus on the task of reaching a solution. Collaboration is needed in order to move nursing forward. Nurses must take an active role in gathering date for evidence-based practice to support the role of nursing in health care and must share this information with other nurses and health professionals.

105. B: Autonomy and self-determination should be viewed within the broad context of diverse cultures. The idea of individualism is less important in some cultures, so the case manager must respect and appreciate the client's right to be guided by her family. Trying to convince the client to assert herself may just lead to emotional conflict. This is not an appropriate concern for the ethics committee, as the woman is not being forced to comply with family decisions but chooses to do so.

106. B: EMTALA prohibits client dumping from EDs. Stabilization of emergent conditions or active labor must be done prior to transfer, and the client's condition should not deteriorate during transfer. **HIPAA** addresses the rights of the individual related to privacy of health information. **ADA** is civil rights legislation that provides the disabled, including those with mental impairment, access to employment and the community. **OAA** provides improved access to services for older adults and Native Americans, including community services (meals, transportation, home health care, adult day care, legal assistance, and home repair).

107. C: The abbreviation of U for units is on the "Do Not Use" list. Other prohibited abbreviations/symbols include IU; QD; QOD; MS, MSO, and MgSO4 for morphine or magnesium sulfate; and trailing zeros (4.0 mg) and lack of a leading zero (.4 mg). Additional abbreviations/symbols are allowed but under consideration for future prohibition. These include <, >, @, cc, μg, and abbreviations of drug names (such as TCN for tetracycline). Using the correct word or term is always better than using an abbreviation, which may be misunderstood, especially if the handwriting is not clear.

108. B: This is an example of **selection bias** because those with catheters without clinically evident infections are excluded. The results are skewed because many clients may have subclinical infections. **Information bias** occurs when there are errors in classification, so an estimate of association is incorrect. Information bias may be nondifferential or differential. **Compliance bias** occurs when adherence to protocol is inconsistent. **Admission bias** occurs when some groups, such as spinal cord injury clients, are omitted from the study.

109. A: The NPSGs requirement for telephone orders or reporting requires that after the information is received and documented, the receiver "read back" the information to ensure that it was heard and documented correctly. Other communication requirements include using a list of approved abbreviations and avoiding unclear or ambiguous abbreviations, acronyms, symbols, or dose designations. Reporting should be done in a timely manner, and the organization should have a standardized manner of hands-off communication that allows for a time to ask/answer questions.

110. C: Clients/family should be apprised of all reasonable risks and any complications that might be life threatening or increase morbidity as well as benefits. The American Medical Association has established the following guidelines for informed consent:

- Explanation of diagnosis.
- Nature and reason for treatment or procedure.
- Risks and benefits.
- Alternative options (regardless of cost or insurance coverage).
- Risks and benefits of alternative options.
- Risks and benefits of not having a treatment or procedure.
- Providing informed consent is a requirement of all states.

111. B: Client safety should always be the primary concern for risk management. Reduction of financial risks and liability relate directly to client safety. A risk management plan should include:

- Goals: Specific and measurable.
- Program scope: Should include linkage with other programs.
- Line of authority: Beginning with the governing board and ending with employees.
- Policies: This should include confidentiality and conflict of interest.
- Data sources and referrals: Types of measures.
- Documentation/reporting: The responsibility for reporting should be clarified and the frequency of reports.
- Activities integration.
- Evaluation of program: The method and frequency of evaluation.
- Charts/diagrams: Flow charts, organizational charts, and diagrams.

112. D: The **Mini-Cog Test** to assess for dementia has two components:

- Drawing the face of a clock with all 12 numbers and the hands indicating the time specified by the examiner.
- Remembering and later repeating the names of three common objects.

The **Mini-Mental State Exam** includes:

- Remembering and later repeating the names of three common objects.
- Counting backward from 100 by 7s or spelling "world" backward.
- Naming items.
- Providing the address and location of the examiner.
- Repeating common phrases.
- Copying a picture of interlocking shapes.
- Following simple three-part instructions.

113. A: Outcomes are derived from client, nurse, and system:

- **Client**: Trust in the healthcare provider based on perceived caring and competency is an essential outcome and links with the functional ability of the client and the quality of life.
- **Nurse**: Measurable outcomes are associated with nursing and include physiological changes, occurrence or prevention of infection, and effectiveness of nursing care and treatments.
- **System**: Outcomes relate to the delivery of care that is consistently both high quality and cost-effective. This includes data regarding rates of rehospitalization, length of hospitalization, and optimal utilization of resources linked to cost data.

114. B: The **home health agency** provides medical and personal care to clients who are homebound and unable to care for themselves. **Public health departments** offer vaccinations and various clinics. Nurses may visit people with communicable diseases, such as tuberculosis, but they do not provide general medical or personal care. **Social services** agencies have social workers who can evaluate people's ability to remain independent, determine if abuse is occurring, and help provide financial support for the needy. **Senior citizens'** organizations vary widely but usually offer social services, such as classes and activities.

115. A: The primary focus of a risk mitigation program is to decrease adverse patient outcomes and reduce liability, so it involves identifying potential risks, such as patient safety issues, and resolving these before they result in litigation or excess costs. Risk mitigation programs usually derive from adverse effects identified retrospectively by risk management. Examples of risk mitigation programs include deep vein thrombosis (DVT) prophylaxis, infection control surveillance, review of patient flow activities, hand hygiene, methicillin-resistant *Staphylococcus aureus* (MRSA) screening, and pressure ulcer prevention programs.

116. B: The **Occupational Safety and Health Administration (OSHA)**, under the Department of Labor, is responsible for bloodborne pathogens standards as well as other workplace standards and inspection of workplaces to ensure safety standards are met. The **Centers for Disease Control and Prevention (CDC)** provides treatment guidelines and recommendations and monitors public health, compiling statistics regarding reportable disease. The **Environmental Protection Agency (EPA)** is not a statutory agency but provides information about the environment to other governmental agencies. The **Food and Drug Administration (FDA)** is a consumer protection agency ensuring safety of medications, biological products, medical devices, and food.

117. A: CQI emphasizes the organization, systems, and processes within that organization rather than individuals. It recognizes internal customers (staff) and external customers (clients) and utilizes data to improve processes, recognizing that most processes can be improved. CQI uses the scientific method of experimentation to meet needs and improve services and utilizes various tools, such as brainstorming, multivoting, various charts and diagrams, storyboarding, and meetings. Core concepts include:

- Quality and success are defined by meeting or exceeding internal and external customers' needs and expectations.
- Problems relate to processes, and variations in process lead to variations in results.
- Change can be incremental.

118. B: Staff preference is subjective and is the weakest justification for establishing a procedure. **Evidence review** includes review of literature, critical analysis of studies, and summarizing of results, including pooled meta-analysis. **Expert judgment**, recommendations based on personal experience from a number of experts, may be utilized, especially if there is inadequate evidence based on review, but this subjective evidence should be explicitly acknowledged. **Policy considerations** include cost-effectiveness, access to care, insurance coverage, availability of qualified staff, and legal implications.

119. D: Viatical settlements benefit the policyholders of life insurance policies. A policyholder essentially sells the policy to a third party so the policyholder can obtain cash to use for care. Beneficiaries must sign a release. HIPAA waives taxes if the policyholder's life expectancy is <24 months, but there may be state or local taxes. Added income may result in interfere with Medicaid benefits. Up to 6 weeks may be necessary before settlements are completed, so those with a very short life expectancy may not benefit.

120. D: An **EPO** provides services at discounted rates to those enrolled. An **HMO** provides a prepaid contract between healthcare providers, payors, and enrollees for specified services in a specified time period, provided by a list of providers. A **POS** is a combination HMO and PPO structure so that people can receive service in the network but can opt to seek treatment outside the network in some situations. **PPOs** involve healthcare providers who have agreed to be part of a network providing services to an enrolled group at reduced rates of reimbursement. Care received outside the network is usually only partially paid for.

121. C: HMO models:

- **Staff:** The HMO hires physicians to work in clinic-type settings. This cost-effective method limits access.
- **Group:** The HMO contracts with multispecialty physician groups, allowing the client more choices.
- **IPA:** The HMO contracts with an independent practice association (IPA) to provide physicians in various specialties. These physicians may see non-HMO clients as well.
- **Network:** The HMO contracts with different physicians and groups in various locations to improve access.
- **Direct contact:** The HMO contracts directly with physicians to provide services rather than through an IPA.

122. C: Medicare B benefits include:

- Clinical laboratory services.
- Medical expenses, including doctor, surgical, and medical services/supplies including durable medical equipment and various therapies (speech, physical, occupational).
- Home health care.
- Outpatient hospital treatment, including diagnostic tests and treatment, ambulatory surgery, mental health services, ambulance services, and administration of blood products.

Medicare A benefits include hospitalization (acute care) with all necessary hospital services and supplies, skilled nursing facility care, hospice care, and administration of blood products.

123. D: Capitation is a healthcare reimbursement system in which providers receive fixed monthly payments in advance of services, based on a negotiated rate. Capitation rates may vary widely. **Pay-for-performance** reimbursement is a system in which providers receive cash incentives to meet specific outcomes (such as reduced infections). **Per-diem reimbursement** provides a fixed daily dollar amount for services, regardless of actual costs. Different types of services may receive different per-diem rates. **Fee-for-service reimbursement** is the traditional system in which providers bill for series provided. This is the most costly type of reimbursement.

124. A: Prevention QIs measure the quality of care for disorders (such as diabetes and heart disease) sensitive to outpatient care, with good care reducing the risk of complications and the need for hospitalization. **Inpatient QIs** measure the quality of care within a hospital and include morbidity and mortality rates for different disorders, utilization of procedures, and volumes of procedures. **PSIs** measure complications and adverse events in hospitals related to surgery, procedures, and labor and delivery. **Pediatric QIs** measure adverse effects of healthcare exposure in the pediatric population.

125. C: CMS core measures include three measures concerning asthma care for children (not adults): relievers (age related), corticosteroids (age related), and plan of care for home management. Additional core measures include eight measures to utilize for care of heart attacks, four measures to care for heart failure, seven measures to care for pneumonia, and five measures to prevent surgical infections. Core measures include standardized procedures to improve the quality of care in hospitals by focusing on outcomes. Hospitals are evaluated based on the percentage rate of compliance.

126 A: URAC (formerly Utilization Review Accreditation Commission) in conjunction with the Case Management Society of America (CMSA) developed case management accreditation standards that require healthcare organizations, such as managed care programs, to establish processes to assess, plan, and implement case management interventions. Categories for assessment include staff structure and organization, staff management/development, quality improvement processes, case management processes, delegation oversight, ethics, and complaint procedures. Policies must be in place to protect the rights of the clients, such as policies for informed consent, conflict resolution, and confidentiality.

127. D: The NCQA administers the Healthcare Effectiveness Data and Information Set (HEDIS) to measure performance of healthcare plans and to help identify plans that provide competent care. NCAQ collects data to demonstrate comparability and consistency in various health plans. Accreditation categories include quality improvement, physician credentials, members' rights/responsibilities, preventive services utilization management, and medical records. HEDIS categories include effectiveness of care, accessibility and availability of care, satisfaction, cost of care, informed decision making, use of services, plan description, and health plan stability.

128. A: The Food and Drug Administration, Code of Federal Regulations, Title 21, Volume 1, regulates **protection of human subjects** and states that any researcher involving clients in research must obtain informed consent, in language understandable to the client or the client's agent. The elements of this informed consent must include an explanation of the research, the purpose, and the expected duration as well as a description off any potential risks. Potential benefits must be described and possible alternative treatments. The client must be informed that participation is voluntary and that he/she can discontinue participation at any time without penalty.

129. D: Supplemental Security Income (SSI) is additional money paid each month to those who are over 65, blind, or disabled with low incomes and few resources. Recipients are allowed only to own their homes and a car, have $1500 in funds set aside for burial and $2000 (single) or $3000 (couple) in savings. While chronic pain may be associated with a disability, pain alone does not qualify the person unless it results in disability that severely impairs function, may result in death, and has been or is expected to persist for 12 months or more.

130. D: Medicaid programs are administered by individual states, which establish eligibility and reimbursement guidelines, so benefits vary considerably from one state to another. Medicaid is a combined federal and state welfare program authorized by Title XIX of the Social Security Act to assist people with low income with payment for medical care. This program provides assistance for all ages, including children. Older adults receiving SSI are eligible as are others who meet state eligibility requirements.

131. B: In the chronic care model, community resources promote the essential element of self-management in conjunction with health systems and organizations, which provide a system of delivery, decision support, and clinical information systems. These work together to allow interactions between an informed client and a proactive team to improve client outcomes. Improved outcomes may include reducing the need for rehospitalization, identifying and anticipating client needs, and reducing costs.

132. C: Out-of-pocket costs are 20%. Medicare, a federal health insurance program for those who have Social Security or bought into Medicare, provides payment to private healthcare providers, such as physicians and hospitals, but limits reimbursement. Physicians receive 80% of usual customary and reasonable (UCR) fees if they accept Medicare assignment. If they do not, they can charge up to 115% of what Medicare allows. Clients are responsible for the remaining 20% or up to 115% if their physicians do not accept Medicare.

133. D: Those eligible for both Tricare and Veterans' Affairs (VA) programs may receive care at VA medical facilities if the service is covered under Tricare and the facility is part of the Tricare network, but the VA cannot bill Medicare, so costs not covered by Tricare must be paid by the client. For those with Medicare, Tricare becomes the secondary insurer. If clients opt out of Medicare, Tricare pays the amount equivalent to a secondary insurer (20% of allowable), and the client is responsible for the rest. By law, all other insurances must pay before Tricare.

134. A: Criteria for Social Security Disability Insurance (SSDI) include a physical/mental disability, which may be temporary (at least 12 months) or permanent (until death) but restricts the person's ability to be gainfully employed. SSDI is available for people under age 65. While SSI has income requirements, SSDI does not. People younger than age 22 may receive SSDI based on parent's work credits, but most people must have accumulated at least 20 Social Security credits over the preceding 10 years for those up to age 42 for eligibility. Those older than age 42 must have one additional Social Security credit for each year of age.

135. B: Out-of-pocket expenses include a **copayment**, which is a specified dollar amount a client must pay at the time of receiving healthcare services, such as a fee of $20 for each physician visit. A **premium** is the monthly cost of an insurance plan. **Coinsurance** is a secondary insurance policy to cover expenses not covered by the primary insurance, such as supplementary insurance plans used in addition to Medicare. A **deductible** is a specified dollar amount that must be paid each year before the insurance plan covers costs, such as a $150 annual deduction.

136. D: The case manager should begin by questioning the reasons for noncompliance to determine the most effective course of action. If the parents are clearly negligent, then a referral to CPS may be indicated, but often noncompliance relates to lack of education about the disease or treatments or lack of adequate financial resources. If caregivers work and the child is expected to do treatments independently, or the child is left with a sitter unfamiliar with the treatment regimen or necessity of maintaining the regimen, then these factors may result in unintentional noncompliance.

137. A: An affidavit of merit is usually filed to support a lawsuit for malpractice. In most states, it must be filed at the time the lawsuit is filed or shortly afterward. A person in the same profession as the defendant swears under oath that there is reasonable cause to proceed and that the evidence suggests that the lawsuit will be successful. This professional may or may not be the same person who provides expert witness testimony during the trial.

138. D: A skilled nursing/rehabilitation facility is the most appropriate placement. Unless the client develops complications, continued therapy in the acute hospital is costly and unnecessary. Home rehabilitation is not appropriate at this stage of recovery because the client lives alone and will still need help with ADLs and exercises. Rehabilitation in a provider office is not appropriate because the client should not yet be alone and has probably not learned to transfer in and out of a vehicle at this early date and would need transportation assistance.

139. A: An ABI score of 0.37 (<0.4) indicates a limb-threatening condition, with pain at rest:

Ankle-brachial index score

>1.3	Abnormally high; may indicate calcification of vessel wall
0.9-1.3	Normal reading; asymptomatic
0.4-0.9	Mild to moderate PAD (narrowing of one or more leg blood vessels) <0.8 is often associated with intermittent claudication during exercise
<0.4	Severe disease and ischemia; pain is present even at rest; limb threatened
<0.25	Critical limb-threatening condition

140. C: Recovery for a person with a chronic mental health disorder means that the client is able to cope with symptoms and problems. In most cases, some symptoms will persist, and clients may still need the intervention of mental health services and may never achieve complete independence in meeting individual needs. The goal of recovery is to allow the client to function to the best of his/her ability with the least amount of supervision and intervention.

141. A: Client empowerment requires that the client have options, so whenever possible the case manager should present more than one choice when decisions must be made. The second requirement is the authority to make decisions. In many cases, clients may assume that the authority lies with others in the healthcare system and don't realize that they have the ultimate authority. The last requirement is action. The case manager should support clients in making decisions about their own care.

142. B: Psychological abuse includes threats and intimidations. Caregivers may make frequent threats to hit the person, sometimes brandishing a weapon if the person doesn't cooperate. Ongoing intimidation may make the person terrified and anxious. Sometimes, caregivers threaten to injure pets or family members, increasing the person's fear. **Physical abuse** includes various types of assaults related to hitting, biting, kicking, pulling hair, shoving, and pushing. **Financial abuse** can include fraud, outright stealing, and forcing people to sign away property. **Neglect**, failure to provide basic needs, may be active/intentional or passive/unintentional.

143. D: Medication reconciliation should be an ongoing process during all phases of care. Medication reconciliation includes making a list of all current medications (dose and frequency), including herbs and OTC drugs and vitamins, as well as drug allergies or intolerances. This list should be posted prominently in the patient's chart so physicians can check the list whenever ordering medications. The patient must receive a new/revised list on discharge with thorough explanation of any changes and access to drug information and the advice of a pharmacist.

144. C: As a mandatory reporter, the case manager should notify appropriate state authorities, such as adult protective services, of the probability of elder abuse. Additional steps, such as notifying the physician or facility owner or even transferring the client, may be necessary to ensure the health and safety of the client, depending on the extent of abuse or neglect. Reprimanding the caregivers may result in their "punishing" the client and may be directed at the wrong caregivers unless the case manager has directly observed abuse.

145. D: Discharge documentation should note improvements related to symptoms or findings present on admission, so "WBC 7,000 and temperature 37 °C" provides the most specific information regarding the change in condition. General statements, such as "stable" and "within normal limits" should be avoided. Discharge documentation is especially important if clients need to be readmitted, as this may become an issue for risk management as it may reflect poor quality of care or too early discharge for status.

146. D: Critical pathways provide a tool for patient management that reduces variations in care. Critical pathways are diagnosis-, procedure-, or condition-specific care plans developed for multiple disciplines, outlining steps in care and expected outcomes. The pathways outline goals in patient care as well as the sequence and time of interventions to achieve those goals. They may be developed for physician care or nursing care. Increasingly, critical pathways are being developed as a method to improve and standardize care and decrease hospital stays.

147. C: The first step in negotiation for a case manager should be research to determine current market values and utilization. The case manager must go to negotiations prepared with facts and figures. Aggressively starting with financial limits or demands about costs is counterproductive, especially if they are unrealistic. Once research is completed, then the case manager can give a statement of the problem and the elements needed to solve the problem (such as the need for physical therapy at a SNF). Clear, honest, open communication is essential. After an agreement is attained, the resolution should be placed in writing and signed by all participants.

148. A: A private case manager is contracted by an individual, family, or insurance company to manage healthcare needs and services. Private case managers represent the company or individual that hires them and try to meet those needs within an ethical framework. When representing an individual, the case manager may assist the transition along the continuum of care and monitor services and outcomes. Private case managing is a form of external (non-hospital-based) management. Independent case managers work for independent case management firms rather than individuals or companies directly.

149. A: General recovery guidelines can be used with clients with very complex medical situations that do not fit into other guidelines. Milliman guides cover a wide range of topics for different levels of care. The guidelines provide specific information needed by case managers to determine if care is appropriate. For example, the coronary artery bypass graft (CABG) guideline provides detailed information about needs: preoperative, acute, recovery facility, home, and risk factor reduction as well as lists of interventions and equipment needed on days one to four.

150. C: Norming. Tuckman's group development stages:

- **Forming**: Leader lists the goals and rules and encourages communication among the members.
- **Storming**: This stage involves a divergence of opinions regarding management, power, and authority. Storming may involve increased stress and resistance as shown by absence, shared silence, and subgroup formation.
- **Norming**: Members express positive feelings toward each other and feel deeply attached to the group.
- **Performing**: The leader's input and direction decreases and mainly consists of keeping the group on course.
- **Mourning**: This is common in closed groups when discontinuation nears and in open groups when the leader or other members leave.

151. C: If a client recently discharged from rehabilitation for substance abuse calls the case manager crying and states she is going to kill herself, the best response is to keep the client on the line and ask another individual to call 9-1-1. It's important to keep the client talking and to encourage the client to talk about her distress and the reasons she is feeling suicidal. Engaging the client can help to defuse the situation until first responders can arrive.

152. B: If a mental health client must attend court-ordered Alcoholics Anonymous® (AA) meetings but tells the case manager that it's a waste of his time and that he is only going because he is forced to because he doesn't have a drinking problem, the most appropriate response is, "It's good that you are attending regularly." This provides positive feedback for what the client is actually doing without challenging the client's insistence that he has no drinking problem.

153. A: If the case manager is evaluating the facility's assessments and polices for fall risks in response to a suit against the facility for a client injury, this type of indicator the case manager is researching is a clinical indicator because it relates to nursing practices and client care. A clinical indicator is a measure to evaluate the quality of client care and to determine if modifications in practice are needed to ensure quality care and client safety.

154. D: Client gender is a factor that is not generally part of caseload calculation although in some instances, the case manager may be serving a population of only one gender (such as pregnant women). A number of different software programs are available to help to calculate caseload. Factors often considered include client acuity, risk stratifications, practice setting, type of record keeping required, type of supervision, and type of care management in addition to any other responsibilities that the case manager may have.

155. B: When considering the cost effectiveness of case management, soft savings can include a client who loses weight and controls diabetes, resulting in fewer emergency room visits. With soft savings, it's not possible to calculate a specific dollar amount of savings because it's impossible to know exactly how many emergency department visits the client would have made if the client had not made changes. However, a review of past records can give some indication of savings. Hard savings are those in which a dollar amount can be calculated, such as with a transfer from an acute care hospital to a skilled nursing facility.

156. B: If a client is transferred from an acute care hospital to an inpatient rehabilitation center, the client must be able to participate in therapy for a minimum of 3 hours daily. The type of therapy may vary but may include speech therapy, occupational therapy, and physical therapy. Clients may also have access to counselors, nutritionists, and social workers. Length of stay varies but is usually 10 to 14 days although some clients will need a longer stay.

157. A: If a 56-year-old client has recovered well from a heart attack and is to undergo cardiac rehabilitation, the best option for the client is likely an outpatient rehabilitation program. The goal of cardiac rehabilitation is preventive, to lower the risk of further cardiac problems. In addition to physical exercise to increase aerobic capacity, increase strength, and improve flexibility, the client may receive additional services, such as nutritional guidance and smoking cessation.

158. B: If a 46-year-old client with cerebral palsy receiving SSDI and Medicare has not worked for pay for 8 years but is interested in doing computer work from home using assistive devices, the case manager should advise the client that he should apply to the Ticket to Work program. This is a government program that provides vocational rehabilitation to clients ages 18 to 64 who are receiving Social Security disability payments. Clients can retain Medicare for up to 93 months, and expedited reinstatement is available for up to 5 years.

159. C: Adult dental care is not one of the 10 essential benefits that must be covered each year by insurance companies without a dollar cap although dental care must be provided for pediatric clients. The 10 essential benefits include ambulatory patient/outpatient services, emergency services, hospitalization, maternity and newborn care, prescriptions drugs, laboratory services, mental health and substance abuse services, rehabilitation and habilitative services/equipment, preventive and wellness/chronic disease services, pediatric services, including oral and vision care.

160. A: If the case manager's laptop computer with FIPS140-2 encryption was stolen and contained PHI regarding clients, the case manager should gather documents proving encryption. FIPS-140-2 is HIPAA compliant encryption and renders the PHI inaccessible, so the loss of the computer does not require a notification of breach; however, the organization should conduct a risk assessment, including reviewing documentation regarding encryption and policies regarding storage of laptops, which should generally be stored in a locked trunk out of the line of sight.

161. D: The situation that is not covered by the Family and Medical Leave Act is a sibling who wants family leave to care for the client during a serious illness. FMLA does not extend benefits to extended family, such as grandparents, in-laws, and siblings, only close family members, such as parents, children, and spouse. FMLA provides those who are eligible up to 12 work weeks of unpaid leave each year, during which time group health benefits must be maintained. The individual must be able to return to the same or an equivalent position after leave. If caring for a service member with serious illness or injury, 26 weeks are allowed in a single year.

162. B: If the client chooses to forego transfer to an inpatient rehabilitation center and have home health care instead against the advice of the physician and the case manager, and the case manager alters the plan of care to correspond with the client's wishes, the case manager is exhibiting the ethical principle of autonomy. The case manager is respecting the client's wishes and doing what the client feels is best while respecting the right of the client to exercise autonomy.

163. C: If a deaf client who prefers to use sign language but can read and type is in a rehabilitation center away from family and friends, the best way for them to communicate is via video chat (Facetime, Skype) because it allows for more natural exchange of ideas. The teletypewriter is another option as are email and messaging, but these choices slow communication and require more effort than video chatting, which is now readily available if the client has access to a smart phone, tablet, or computer.

164. B: When documenting a verbal exchange with a client, the case manager must avoid subjective opinions and provide an objective report: "Client states treatment is not working and, therefore, refused to take medications." Whenever possible, the reason for the client's action should be included, not just that the client is refusing treatment, because the information that the client believes the treatment is ineffective is important for healthcare workers to address with the client.

165. C: When considering whether the Americans with Disabilities Act will provide protections for a client, the case manager recognizes that a condition that is not considered a disability is transsexualism. While the ADA does not provide an exclusive list of covered conditions, generally, conditions related to addictions (drugs, gambling) are not covered, nor are conditions related to sexual preferences or differences, such as homosexuality, transsexualism, and transvestism. However, transsexuals are protected in the workplace by the Civil Rights Act.

166. A: The case manager uses Interqual®, an evidence-based tool, in order to determine the client's level of acuity and level of care needed. Interqual® offers a number of products: Levels of care criteria, Care planning criteria, behavioral health criteria, coordinated care content, and evidence-based development. The goals of Interqual® include preventing over- and under-utilization, reducing risks, facilitating communication, improving data collection, supporting consistency of care in alignment with CMS guidelines, reducing costs, identifying areas in which improvement can be made, facilitating payments, and identifying trends.

167. D: The assessment that must be included in the Inpatient Rehabilitation Facility Patient Assessment Instrument (IRF-PAI) for CMS to determine the rate of payment for fee-for-service clients is the Functional Independence Measure™ (FIM™). This tool evaluates the client's level of disability. Admission scores are obtained during the first three days of rehabilitation hospitalization based on observations over the entire 3-day period. FIM™ items include eating, grooming, bathing, upper dressing, lower dressing, toileting, bladder, bowel, transfers (bed, chair, wheelchair), transfers (toilet), transfers (tub/shower), walk/wheelchair, stairs, comprehension, expression, social interaction, problem solving, and memory.

168. D: If the case manager is utilizing the strengths model of case management, the case manager must assist the client to identify abilities, skills, and environmental factors that may promote recovery. The strengths model of case management focuses on client's strengths rather than deficits in planning interventions based on the belief that people have inner resources that can help them to cope. The relationship between the case manager and the client is considered essential. Clients' problems are viewed in the context of goals, and methods are developed to overcome the problems rather than viewing them as barriers to recovery.

169. C: Accommodation. Approaches to negotiation include:

Competition	One party wins and the other loses.
Accommodation	One party concedes to the other; the losing side may gain little or nothing.
Avoidance	Negotiation is avoided and nothing is resolved; likely when both parties dislike conflict.
Compromise	Both parties make concessions in order to reach a consensus; this can result in decisions that satisfy no one.
Collaboration	The parties work together to arrive at a solution that provides everyone with a satisfactory result; a win-win solution and often a creative one.

170. D: If an Inpatient Prospective Patient System hospital is in the Hospital Readmissions Reduction Program, the hospital is penalized by being reimbursed at a lower rate if a client has an unplanned readmission for a condition included in the program within 30 days or for a client who is admitted to the same or any acute care hospital for any reason with 30 days. Planned readmissions are not counted against the facility. A payment adjustment factor is calculated for each eligible hospital.

171. B: If a client with repeated emergency department visits for migraine headaches has received relief from a new treatment, but the client's insurance does not yet cover the cost of the very expensive medication and denied an appeal, the case manager should advise the client to apply to the pharmaceutical company's patient assistance program. Such programs often supply the drug at lowered cost or free for up to a year. New treatments are often denied by insurance companies until more data are available.

172. A: If the case manager is utilizing video calls with clients rather than in-person visits, the HIPAA regulations regarding privacy and security must apply. Therefore, the video calls must be encrypted so that the calls cannot be accessed by others. The Privacy rule protects any information in the medical record, billing information, conversations between the client and case manager, and other health information. The security rule requires that electronic health information be secure and protected and safeguards be in place.

173. C: With the disease management model of case management, the case manager focuses on post-acute services for chronic illness to reduce readmissions. Typical clients include those with COPD, heart disease, liver disease, renal disease, and diabetes. Case management may include educating clients about their disease, and proving guidance in making lifestyle changes (weight loss, increased exercise, smoking cessation) and in better managing of disease. Additionally, the case manager may assist the client to access community resources, such as Meals-on-Wheels and low-cost transportation services.

174. D: If the case manager is part of an interdisciplinary team in which two members of the team have a disagreement regarding client care, the first step to resolving the conflict is to allow both individuals to present their side of the disagreement without bias, keeping the focus on the opinions rather than the individuals. Often, individuals just want to feel that they are heard and their views are appreciated. Then, the case manager should encourage the individual to cooperate with negotiation and compromise.

175. A: The case manager's primary role in transitions of care is to ensure that the client receives the appropriate level of care and services. The client's status should be assessed on a daily basis to determine if stepdown (such as from ICU to a medical-surgical unit) or transfer to another facility (such as a skilled nursing facility) is indicated because overutilization can result in decreased pay for services. Even though there are financial incentives to appropriate transitions of care, this should not be the primary factor for case management.

176. B: In terms of utilization management, and example of underutilization is if the hospital lacks an MRI and must transfer clients needing an MRI to another hospital. Trends that are analyzed as part of utilization management include:

- Overutilization: This may relate to inappropriate admissions, levels of care, length of stay, or undocumented rationale for resource use (such as lab tests).
- Underutilization: Level of care or resources may be inadequate for medical necessity (failure to admit, inadequate testing).
- Misutilization: This includes errors in treatment or other inefficiencies, such as scheduling.

177. D: According to Lewin's force field analysis of change, a driving force would be competition. Force field analysis includes:

- Driving forces: These are forces responsible for instigating and promoting change, such as leaders, incentives, and competition.
- Restraining forces: These are forces that resist change, such as poor attitudes, hostility, inadequate equipment, or insufficient funds.

Force field analysis is used when considering changes and begins by listing a proposed change and creating two subgroups below: driving and restraining forces. In order to bring about change, a plan must be developed to diminish or eliminate the restraining forces.

178. B: As part of a wellness program, clients with average risk should begin colorectal screening at age 50. Those with increased risk, should begin screening at age 40. Increased risk factors include:

- Family history of colorectal cancer in first or second-degree relatives.
- Family history of genetic syndrome (FAP, HNLPCC).
- Adenomatous polyps in first-degree relatives before age 60.
- History of polyps or colorectal cancer.
- History of inflammatory bowel disease.

Screening may include fecal occult blood, flexible sigmoidoscopy, colonoscopy, capsule colonoscopy, and/or double contrast barium enema.

179. D: Preparation. Transtheoretical stages:

- Precontemplation: Client informed about consequences of problem behavior and has no intention of changing behavior in the next 6 months.
- Contemplation: Client aware of costs and benefits of changing behavior and intends to change in the next 6 months but is procrastinating.
- Preparation: Client has a plan to instigate change in the near future (≤1 month) and is ready for action plans.
- Action: Client modifies behavior. Change occurs only if behavior meets a set criterion (such as complete abstinence from drinking).
- Maintenance: Client works to maintain changes and gains confidence that he/she will not relapse.

180. A: If a 35-year-old client with rheumatoid arthritis has become increasingly withdrawn and socially isolated and states that her family and friends don't understand what she is going through, an appropriate intervention is referral to support group. Clients with chronic illnesses often benefit from participating in a support group with others with the same disease because clients often find that they can express what they are feeling and the challenges they face more freely and gain insight from the group regarding coping strategies.

Thank You

We at Mometrix would like to extend our heartfelt thanks to you, our friend and patron, for allowing us to play a part in your journey. It is a privilege to serve people from all walks of life who are unified in their commitment to building the best future they can for themselves.

The preparation you devote to these important testing milestones may be the most valuable educational opportunity you have for making a real difference in your life. We encourage you to put your heart into it—that feeling of succeeding, overcoming, and yes, conquering will be well worth the hours you've invested.

We want to hear your story, your struggles and your successes, and if you see any opportunities for us to improve our materials so we can help others even more effectively in the future, please share that with us as well. **The team at Mometrix would be absolutely thrilled to hear from you!** So please, send us an email (support@mometrix.com) and let's stay in touch.

If you feel as though you need additional help, please check out the other resources we offer:

Study Guide: http://MometrixStudyGuides.com/CCM

Flashcards: http://MometrixFlashcards.com/CCM